Acupuncture in Clinical Practice

by Drs. Lo Chi Kwong & Tsui Sui King

THE COMMERCIAL PRESS, LTD.

ACUPUNCTURE IN CLINICAL PRACTICE
中國針刺經穴學

by Drs. Lo Chi Kwong & Tsui Sui King
Published by THE COMMERCIAL PRESS, LTD.
4/F., Kiu Ying Building, 2D, Finnie Street,
Quarry Bay, Hong Kong.
Printed by
C & C JOINT PRINTING CO., (H.K.) LTD.
75, Pau Chung Street, Kowloon, Hong Kong.

First Edition January 1979
Reprinted January 1984

ISBN 962 07 3050 X

CONTENTS

Foreword

Following the Ping Pong diplomacy initiated by the Peoples' Republic of China in the early 70's, there has been growing interest in the health care delivery system of China, which emphasizes the integration of Western with traditional Chinese medicine. Peoples of the West are intrigued by the use of acupuncture for the treatment of disease conditions and especially by its use to create analgesia for major surgical operations.

The Chinese Medical Research Center was founded in 1971 with the main aim of promoting the use of Chinese traditional medicine among practitioners of Western medicine. One of its first programmes was to begin a series of training courses of acupuncture for practitioners of Western medicine. Since then its "graduates" are found all over the world.

One of the problems encountered by the Center has been the lack of good instruction material written in the English language. Therefore this new book, compiled by Drs. C.K. Lo & S.K. Tsui, will be a welcome addition, as it was only contains a more detailed description of the Meridians (Jing), Extra-meridians (Mai), and Strange and New points, but also a useful summary on the choice of points in various clinical conditions.

L.K. Ding, MD. MCPS
Chairman and Founder,
Chinese Medical Research Center.

Preface

The theory of Acupuncture is based on the fundamental concepts of Yin and Yang, the Five Elements and the meridians postulated in the Traditional Chinese Medicine.

Acupuncture has been used and developed over the last 2000 years and forms a systematic pattern from accumulated experience, experimentation and observation.

Since acupuncture treatment neither requires any drugs nor produces side effects or habituation; whilst at the same time is highly effective in various disease such as migraine, toothache, trigeminal neuralgia etc, for those trained in western medicine it can, therefore, become an intergral part of the practice modern medicine.

In recent years though many practitioners have considered acupuncture very important, their work has been mainly confined to basic needling methods and points, neglecting the importance of meridians, which forms the basis of the practice of this modality of treatment.

In order to cope with the progress and development of needling methods, this book has been written, hoping that it will be of some help to contemporary acupuncturists.

This book emphasizes the pathways of the meridians

and is divided into four parts:
1. Some basic concepts of traditional Chinese Medicine.
2. The course and direction of each meridian.
3. Organs connected with each meridian and connective points with other meridians.
4. Points commonly used on each meridian along with their indications.

It is only with a sound understanding of the theory of meridians, the five elements and Chinese Medicine, can one really practice the needling method correctly.

The authors of this book is particularly grateful to Dr. L. K. Ding, M.D., Chairman of The Chinese Medical Research Center, who has kindly agreed to write a Foreword to this book. Dr. L. K. Ding has a wide knowledge and experience of both Western medicine as well as the techniques of acupuncture.

(Note: The author of this book has also written a seperate book on three new fields of nose, hand and foot acupuncture field.)

Dr. C.K. Lo & Dr. S.K. Tsui

Chapter 1
History of Acupuncture

In ancient time long before the advent of modern medicine, our ancestors had the practice of using thin sharp stones to prick the body to cure certain disease. Since the results were very good, this practice of body pricking was further explored and developed. The change was first in the instrument. Needles were changed from sharp stones to porcelain then to gold, silver, copper and in more recent years, from stainless steel.

As early as the 21st century B.C., Chinese acupuncture was considered a form of therapy as important as medicine itself and was extremely popular among the common people. The book 'Huang Dei Nei Jing' (The Emperor's Classic of Internal Medicine 黃帝內經 which was written in 400-200 B.C., had already given a description of acupuncture, pointing out the interrelationship between the meridians, moxibustion and their indications for use in disease. This book served as the basis for the further development of acupuncture.

Then in 141-203 A.D., the most famous surgeon of China, Hua To (華陀) used a needle into GB 19 (206)

(Location: lateral side of the occipital protuberance, right above point GB 20) to relief headache for emperor Tsao Tsiao (曹操). He also used points GB 30 (217) (Location: one third distance from the greater trochanter to the sacral hiatus) and GB 39 (226) (Location: three tsun above the lateral malleolus) to relieve pain in his lower extremities. Each treatment produced excellent result.

In 960-1643 A.D., the first copper model, showing all the acupuncture points was made. This model showed the running direction of the meridians and served as the guideline for the further study of acupuncture.

The plastic models we see today are also reproductions of the old copper model. In addition, eight extra meridians (Mai脈) have also been discovered. They are Doe Mai (Governing Vessel), Jei Mai (Conception Vessel), Dai Mai, Yin Wei Mai, Yang Wei Mai, Yin Chiao Mai and Yang Chiao Mai. Through this combination of the old copper model and the new findings, we now have the 12 regular Meridians (Jing 經) and eight extra meridians (Mai 脈).

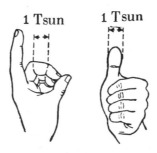

Fig. 1   The Tsun

The Chinese unit of length is the 'Tsun' (寸). It is the width of the patient's thumb at the first interphalangeal joint crease, or the length between the crease of the interphalangeal joint of the middle finger as shown in Fig. 1

The knowledge of acupuncture then spread to foreign countries in the sixth century. The first countries to learn and practice this mode of therapy were Korea and Japan. It was not until Willhelm Ten Rhyme of the East India Company wrote a book on acupuncture that western countries become aware of this art. Since then, France, Germany, America, England, Australia and other countries began using acupuncture as a form of medical treatment. Today, many acupuncture associations are established in various countries, and the development is closely watched by all medical fields concerned.

Chapter 2
The basic theory of Chinese Medicine

It is essential to understand some basic background of the theories of Chinese medicine before we go into the details of the Meridian system. According to the theory of traditional Chinese medicine, channels (Jing and Mei) play a very important part in the field of acupuncture. Besides, "Chi", "Yin", "Yang", and the five elements are the basic concepts for diagnosis and treatment of most diseases.

"Chi" means the "Energy of Life". It has the power to create and to change all matter. It controls the life and death of the human body. In a healthy body, the passage of this "Chi" should be free from obstruction and interruption. It starts from the lungs, and travels through the meridians in a systematic manner.

"Yin" and "Yang" are two matters contained within this "Chi". They are in balance but in opposite pairs. Any imbalance of these will result in sickness. Some of the examples are as follows:—

Yin - Chronic disease, malaise, tuberculosis, solid organs (heart, pericardium, lung, kidney, spleen, liver), the front of the body and medial side of the extremities.

Yang - Pneumonia, acute disease, fever, tachycardia, hollow organs (large intestine, triple warmer, small intestine, stomach, gallbladder, bladder), the back of the body and lateral side of the extremities.

"Yin" and "Yang" do not exist in isolation. They interrelate and interact on each other. If a patient is sick, the acute state may belong to the Yang. However, Yin may also be involved in the later stage. They are never static or absolute. A part of the Yin may exist in Yang and a part of Yang may exist in the Yin. The interplay of the Yin and the Yang is a dynamic one.

The Five Elements in Chinese medicine are composed

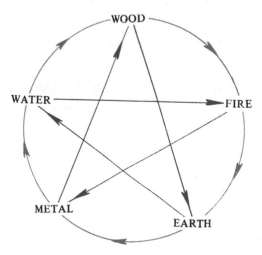

Fig. 2   The Five Elements

Note: — blue colour line indicates the Creative cycle.

— red colour line indicates the Destructive cycle.

of the following matter:— Wood, Fire (major Fire and minor Fire), Earth, Metal and Water. These five elements travel in two different cycles, the Creative cycle or "shen" (生) cycle and the Destructive cycle or "ko" (尅) cycle. (Fig. 2)

In the actual practice of acupuncture, the five elements are related to internal organs and any one part of the body.

Wood corresponds to the liver, gall-bladder, ligament and eyes.

Major fire corresponds to the heart, small intestine, vessel and tongue.

Minor fire corresponds to the pericardium, triple warmer, vessel and tongue.

Earth corresponds to the spleen, stomach, muscle and mouth.

Metal corresponds to the lung, large intestine, skin and nose.

Water corresponds to the kidney, bladder, bone and ear.

Besides the five elements, a channel system is also a main theme in the theory of Chinese medicine. The channel system consists of a regular Meridian (Jing 經) and an extra Meridian (Mai 脈). These channels exist in the form of a network connecting the internal organs and the superficial parts of the body. They are responsible for regulating the function of the whole body.

Meridians (the proper name for Jing 經) travel in a vertical direction within the body. There are altogether 12 pairs meridians. Each with its own definite pathway.

Pathways are classified as internal and external pathways.

For example, the Arm Greater Yin Lung Meridian, which originates in the middle warmer and lung, traverses inside the body and then is linked to the external pathway at the starting point L1 (location: lateral part of the first intercostal space). The end of this external pathway will terminate at L11 (location: radial side of the tip of thumb) and radial side of the index finger, where it is linked to another meridian — the Arm Sunlight Yang Large Intestine Meridian, which relates to the large intestine.

Therefore, the whole channel system is a closed circuit one, the route having a definite direction of flow. This closed circuit system is the basis of cure effected by inserting a needle at a certain point along this system of channel. For example, when a needle is inserting into point S 36 it should cure indigestion and gastritis, since this point, S 36 is linked to the stomach and spleen (according to the theory of Chinese medicine, the function of spleen and stomach are the same). Therefore, any stimulation given to the leg at S 36 will create an effect on the viscera, through the related meridian.

The following are some general concepts of meridians:

The 12 pairs of meridians are sysmetrically distributed bilaterally over the entire body. They are named according to Yin or Yang, Arm or Leg and their related Organ.

There are six pairs of meridians in the upper extremities. (Fig. 3)

Ventral side of Upper Extremities:

Meridian	Location
Heart Meridian	Ulnar side
Pericardium Meridian	Middle
Lung Meridian	Radial side

These pairs run from chest to hand.

Dorsal side of Upper Extremities:

Meridian	Location
Large Intestine Meridian	Radial side
Triple Warmer Meridian	Middle
Small Intestine Meridian	Ulnar side

These pairs run from the hand to face.

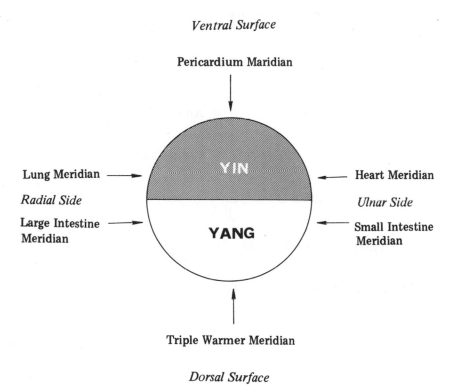

Fig. 3 The Postions Occupied By The Left Upper Limb Meridians

There are also six pairs of meridians in the lower extremities. (Fig. 4)

Lateral side of lower Extremities:

Meridian	Location
Stomach Merdian	Antero-Lateral side
Gall-bladder Meridian	Middle-Lateral
Bladder Meridian	Postero-Lateral side

These pairs run from the face to the feet.

Medial side of Lower extremities:

Meridian	Location
Kidney Meridian	Posteromedial side
Liver Meridian	Medial middle
Spleen Meridian	Anteromedial side

These pairs run from the feet to the chest.

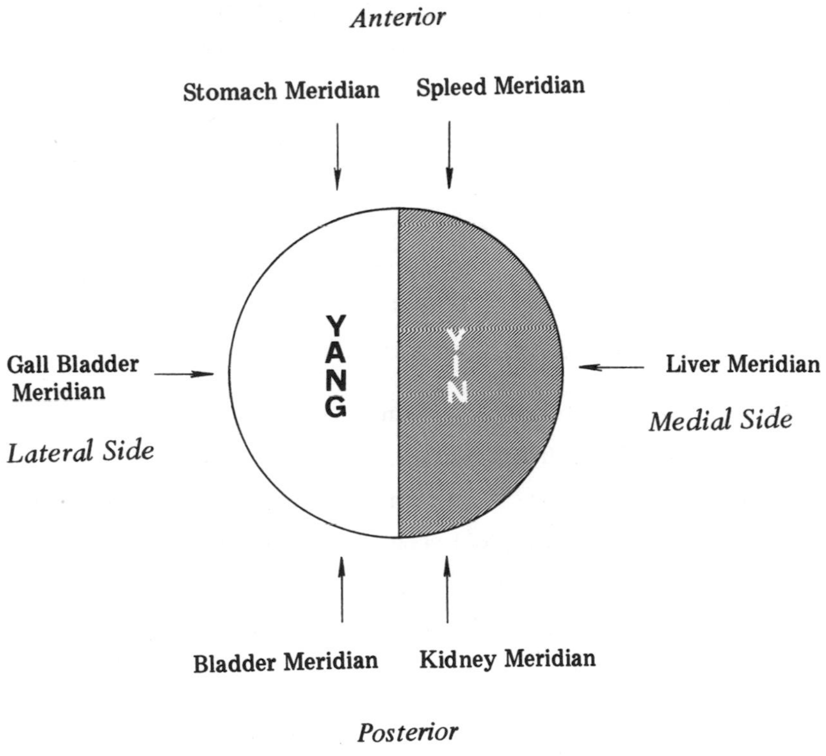

Fig. 4   The Postions Occupied By The Left Lower Limb Meridians

Meridians can be classified as Yin and Yang. There are three kinds of Yin Meridian:

YIN
1. Greater Yin   Arm: — Lung Meridian (L)
    (Tai Yin 太陰)   Leg: — Spleen Meridian (Sp)
2. Lesser Yin   Arm: — Heart Meridian (H)
    (Shao Yin 少陰)   Leg: — Kidney Meridian (K)
3. Absolute Yin   Arm: — Pericardium Meridian (P)
    (Chueh Yin 厥陰) Leg: — Liver Meridian (Liv)
    ( )   Abreviations commonly employed

There are also three kinds of Yang Meridians:

YANG
1. Sunlight Yang   Arm: — Large Intestine Meridian (LI)
    (Yang Ming 陽明) Leg: — Stomach Meridian (S)
2. Lesser Yang   Arm: — Triple Warmer Meridian (TW)
    (Shao Yang 少陽) Leg: — Gall Bladder Meridian (GB)
3. Greater Yang   Arm: — Small Intestine Meridian (SI)
    (Tai Yang 太陽) Leg: — Bladder Meridian (B)
    ( )   Abreviations commonly employed

In fact, all the names given to the meridians are Yin or Yang, Arm or Leg, plus their related internal organ, i.e., the Arm Greater Yin Lung Meridian and the Leg Sunlight Yang Stomach Meridian.

There are eight extra-meridians. They are called the Doe Mai (the governing vessel 督脈) and Jei Mai (the conception vessel 任脈), which are unpaired. In addition,

there are 6 other meridians namely: — Chong Mai (沖脈),
Dai Mai (帶脈), Yin Wei Mai (陰維脈), Yang Wei Mai
(陽維脈), Yin Chiao Mai (陰蹻脈) and Yang Chiao Mai
(陽蹻脈).

The above eight extra-meridians have branches connecting the main meridians. However, they are different from
meridians as they do not belong to any internal organ.

The Governing Vessel connects with three yang
meridians of the arm and leg at point GV 14. The Conception
vessel connect three Yin meridians of the leg at CV 3 and
CV 4.

Chong Mai is connected to the Leg Sunlight Yang
Stomach Meridian, the Leg Lesser Yin Kidney Meridian,
the Governing vessel and the Conception Vessel.

Dai Mai is formed like a belt surrounding the loin
connecting with many meridians which pass through the
waist such as the Governing vessel, the Conception vessel,
the Leg Lesser Yang Gall-Bladder Meridian, etc.

Yang Chiao Mai, Yin Chiao Mai, Yinwei and Yangwei
connect with the Yang and Yin meridian of arm and leg
respectively.

The co-relation between the Yin, Yang and Meridian cycle.

	Yin (Solid organ)		Yang (Hollow organ)		
Greater Yin	Lung	Arm	Large Intestine	Arm	Sunlight Yang
	Spleen	Leg	Stomach	Leg	
Lesser Yin	Heart	Arm	Small Intestine	Arm	Greater Yang
	Kidney	Leg	Bladder	Leg	
Absolute Yin	Pericardium	Arm	Triple Warmer	Arm	Lesser Yang
	Liver	Leg	Gall-Bladder	Leg	

Footnote:— The arrows indicate the flow of 'Chi' from one meridian to another.

The relationship between the Five Elements and Meridian

Yang	Meridian	Arm sunlight Yang	Leg Greater Yang	Leg lesser Yang	Arm Greater Yang	Leg sunlight Yang	Arm lesser Yang
	Organ	Large intestine	Bladder	Gall-Bladder	Small intestine	Stomach	Triple Warmer
Five Elements		Metal	Water	Wood	Major Fire	Earth	Minor Fire
Yin	Meridian	Arm Greater Yin	Leg Lesser Yin	Leg Absolute Yin	Arm Lesser Yin	Leg Greater Yin	Arm Absolute Yin
	Organ	Lung	Kidney	Liver	Heart	Spleen	Pericardium

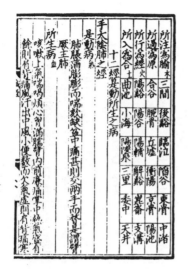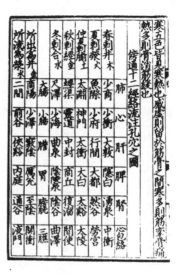

寒五色皆見寒熱也歲盛則留於筋骨之間寒多則筋攣骨痛熱多則骨消筋緩故也

傍通十二經絡流注孔穴之圖

	肺	心	肝	脾	腎	心包絡
春刺井木	少商	少衝	大敦	隱白	湧泉	中衝
夏刺榮火	魚際	少府	行間	大都	然谷	勞宮
仲夏刺腧土	太淵	神門	太衝	太白	太谿	大陵
秋刺經金	經渠	靈道	中封	商丘	復溜	間使
冬刺合水	尺澤	少海	曲泉	陰陵泉	陰谷	曲澤

	大腸	小腸	膽	胃	膀胱	三焦
所出為井金	商陽	少澤	竅陰	厲兌	至陰	關衝
所流為榮水	二間	前谷	俠谿	內庭	通谷	液門
所注為腧木	三間	後谿	臨泣	陷谷	束骨	中渚
所過為原	合谷	腕骨	丘墟	衝陽	京骨	陽池
所行為經火	陽谿	陽谷	陽輔	解谿	崑崙	支溝
所入為合土	曲池	小海	陽陵泉	三里	委中	天井

十二經是動所生之病

手太陰肺之經

是動病 肺脹滿膨膨而喘欬缺盆中痛甚則交兩手而瞀是謂臂厥

所主肺

所生病 欬嗽上氣喘喝煩心胸滿臑臂內前廉痛厥掌中熱氣盛有餘則肩背痛風汗出中風小便數而欠氣虛則肩背痛寒

Fig. 5   The relationship between the meridians and points

16

Chapter 3
The Arm Greater Yin Lung
Meridian and points

I.   The Arm Greater Yin Lung Meridian

There are a total of 11 points on this meridian.

(A)   Direction:

It originates in the middle warmer, goes downwards to the large intestine, then turns back around the cardia, passes up through the diaphragm into the lungs and trachea and at the first intercostal space connects with the external pathway. This superficial branch (External pathway) descends along the radial side of the arm to the radial side of the thumb (Fig. 6, Fig. 7).

(B)   Branches:

There is an internal branch off this meridian. It arises above the styloid process of the radius at L 7 point which runs to the radial side of the tip of the index finger.

(C)   Connected Internal Organs:

Lung, Stomach and Large Intestine.

The termination of this meridian connects with The Arm Sunlight Yang Large Intestine Meridian at the radial side of the tip of the index finger.

(D) Connective points:
   None.

II Points Commonly Used:

L 1 (52)
Location: Lateral side of the first intercostal space, 2 tsun on the medial side of the anterior axillary fold.

Indications: Asthma, Bronchitis, special treatment for Pulmonary diseases.

Method of Insertion: Slanting insertion of 0.5 − 0.8 tsun deep.

L 2 (53)
Location: Below the acromial extremity of the clavicle, right in the infraclavicular fossa.

Indications: Cough, Shoulder Pain, special treatment for upper respiratory tract diseases.

Method of Insertion: A slanting insertion of 0.5 − 1 tsun deep.

L 5 (56)
Location: At the elbow crease on the radial side of the biceps brachii tendon.

Indications: Hemoptysis, Swollen and painful elbow joint.

Method of Insertion: A straight insertion of 1.0 − 1.5 tsun deep.

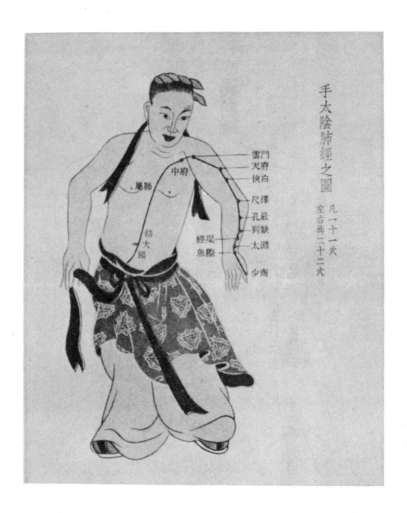

Fig. 6   The Arm Greater Yin Lung Meridian

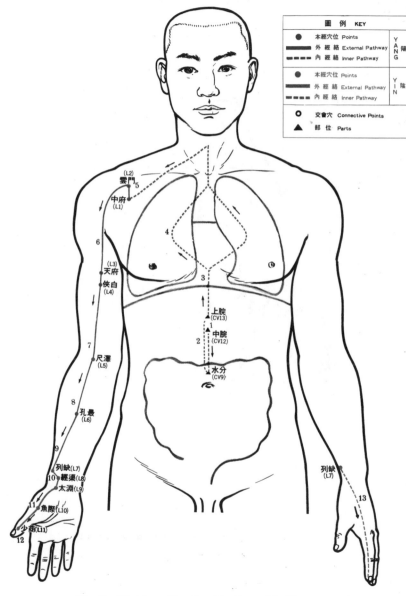

Fig. 7　The Arm Greater Yin Lung Meridian

L 7 (58)

Location: Above the styloid process of the radius, 1.5 tsun above the most distal skin crease of the wrist.

Indications: Headache, wryneck, special treatment for head and nape diseases.

Method of Insertion: A slanting insertion of 0.5 – 1 tsun deep.

L 10 (61)

Location: On the palmer surface, at the middle of the first metacarpal bone.

Indications: Hemoptysis, Fever.

Method of Insertion: A straight insertion of 0.5 tsun deep.

L 11 (62)

Location: 0.1 tsun proximal to the corner of the nail on the radial side of the thumb.

Indications: Epilepsy, Coma, Apoplexy.

Method of Insertion: Straight insertion of 0.1 tsun or use a triangular needle to prick the point and cause a little bleeding.

Chapter 4

The Arm Sunlight Yang Large Intestine Meridian and points

I. The Arm Sunlight Yang Large Intestine Meridian

There are a total of 20 points on this meridian.

(A) Direction:

It starts at the radial side of the tip of the index finger and then ascends to the middle of the first and second metacarpal bone, along the radial side of arm to the shoulder area, at the LI 16 point it connects with the internal pathway pass through the GV 14 point to the supraclavicular fossa. This internal pathway descends to the lung, stomach and large intestine. (Fig. 8, Fig. 9)

(B) Branches:

The first mixed branch: starts from the supraclavicular fossa and goes up to the angle of mandible and upper lip, crossing the Governing Vessel at GV 26 point to the opposite side of ala nasi.

The second internal branch: starts at the lower border of the zygomatic bone, then goes into the lower lip and lower gum.

The third internal branch: starts at the LI 14 point

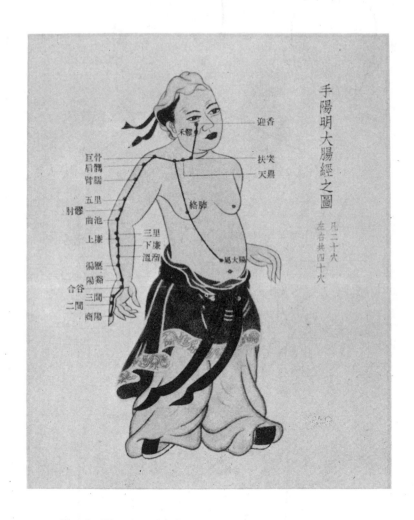

Fig. 8   The Arm Sunlight Yang Large Intestine Meridian

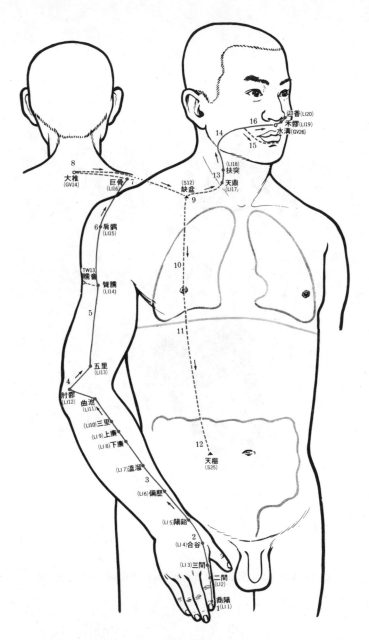

迎香(LI20)
禾髎(LI19)
水溝(GV26)
16
14
15
扶突(LI18)
13 天鼎(LI17)
8
大椎(GV14)
巨骨(LI16)
缺盆(S12)
9
6 肩髃(LI15)
TW13
臑會
臂臑(LI14)
5
10
11
五里(LI13)
4
肘髎(LI12)
曲池(LI11)
三里(LI10)
上廉(LI9)
下廉(LI8)
溫溜(LI7)
3
偏歷(LI6)
12 天樞(S25)
陽谿(LI5)
2
合谷(LI4)
三間(LI3)
二間(LI2)
商陽(LI1)
1

Fig. 9   The Arm Sunlight Yang Large Intestine Meridian

connects with the Arm Lesser Yang Triple Warmer Meridian at TW 13 point.

(C) Connected Internal Organs:

Stomach, Large Intestine, Lung.

(D) Connective Points:

GV 14, GV 26 – connecting the Governing Vessel. S 4 – connecting The Leg Sunlight Yang Stomach Meridian.

The termination of this meridian connects with the Leg Sunlight Yang Stomach Meridian at the side of ala nasi.

II Points Commonly Used:

LI 1 (81)

Location: 0.1 tsun proximal to the corner of nail, on the radial side of the index finger.

Indications: Numbness of finger, Fever, Apoplexy, Pharyngitis.

Method of Insertion: Straight insertion of 0.1 – 0.2 tsun deep with the triangular needle, a little bleeding may be caused.

LI 4 (84)

Location: Between the first and second metacarpal bones at the highest spot of muscle when the thumb and index finger are closed together.

Indications: Headache, Toothache, Bell's Palsy, Hemiplegia, Common cold and fever, special treatment for face, mouth and tooth pain.

Method of Insertion: Straight or slanting insertion of 0.5 tsun to 1 tsun deep.

LI 5 (85)

Location: At the radial side of the back of wrist, between the tendons of extensor pollicis brevis and longus, just over the anatomical snuff box.

Indications: Eye pain, Deafness, Tinnitus, Wrist pain.

Method of Insertion: Straight insertion of 0.3 − 0.5 tsun deep.

LI 7 (87)

Location: 5 tsun above LI 5 (85)

Indications: Arm pain.

Method of Insertion: Straight insertion of 0.5 − 1.0 tsun deep. Slanting insertion of 1.0 − 1.5 tsun deep.

LI 11 (91)

Location: At the external end of the elbow crease.

Indications: Hypertension, Paralysis, Elbow pain.

Method of Insertion: Straight insertion of 1 − 1.5 tsun deep or point to point method towards H3 (74)

LI 14 (94)

Location: 7 tsun above LI 11 (91) at the lower end of the

26

deltoid muscle.

Indications: Arm pain, Hemiplegia.

Method of Insertion: Straight insertion of 0.5 − 1 tsun deep.
Slanting insertion of 1.0 − 1.5 tsun deep.

LI 15 (95)

Location: At the anterio-inferior point of the acromion.

Indications: Frozen shoulder, Hemiplegia.

Method of Insertion: Slanting insertion of 0.5 − 1 tsun deep.

LI 18 (98)

Location: 3 tsun beside the middle of the laryngeal prominence, between the two heads of the sterno-cleido-mastoid muscle.

Indications: Cough, Copious Sputum.

Method of Insertion: Straight insertion of 0.5 − 1 tsun deep.

LI 20 (100)

Location: 0.5 tsun beside the ala nasi.

Indications: Rhinitis, Bell's palsy.

Method of Insertion: Slanting insertion of 0.3 − 0.5 tsun in a medial and upwards direction.

Chapter 5

The Leg Sunlight Yang Stomach
Meridian and points

I.   The Leg Sunlight Yang Stomach Meridian

There are a total of 45 points on this meridian.

(A) Direction:

It starts at the alae nasi, goes to the prominence of the nose connecting with the Leg Greater Yang Bladder Meridian at the medial canthus (B 1 point). Then goes straight down to the angle of the mouth and joins the conception vessel at CV 24. From the mentolabial sulcus, it goes back to the anterior border of the masseteric muscle and ascends to the front part of the ear and then to the angle of the forehead, connecting with the Governing Vessel at GV 24 point. (Fig. 10, Fig. 11)

(B) Branches:

The first external branch — starts from the lower border of mandible, then goes down to the supraclavicular fossa along the lateral side of the chest and abdomen, goes down to the inguinal area and descends to the thigh, leg, to end on the lateral side of the second toe.

The second internal branch — starts at the supraclavicular

fossa through the diaphragm connecting with the stomach and spleen and joins with the first branch on the inguinal region at S 30 point.

The third internal branch — starts at the S 36 point and descends to the lateral side of the third toe.

The fourth internal branch — starts at S 42 point and descends to the big toe.

(C) Connected Internal Organs:

Stomach, Spleen, Heart, Large Intestine and Small Intestine.

(D) Connective Points

LI 20 (the Arm Sunlight Yang Large Intestine Meridian)

B 1 (the Leg Greater Yang Bladder Meridian)

GB 3, GB 4, GB 5, GB 6 (the Leg Lesser Yang Gall-Bladder Meridian)

GV 26, GV 24, GV 14 (Governing Vessel)

CV 24, CV 13, CV 12 (Conception Vessel)

The termination of this meridian connects with the Leg Greater Yin Spleen Meridian at the big toe.

II   Commonly Used Points:

S 1 (143)

Location: Between the eyeball and the inferior border of the orbit.

Indications: Myopia, Optic neuritis, Conjunctivitis.

Method of Insertion: Slanting insertion of 0.3 — 0.5 tsun

deep along the edge of orbit. The
patient is asked to look up. New
method use 1.0 − 1.3 tsun deep.

S 2 (144)

Location: Just over the infra-orbital foramen.

Indications: Bell's palsy, Trigeminal neuralgia.

Method of Insertion: Straight insertion of 0.2 − 0.3 tsun
deep or slanting insertion of 1 − 2.5
tsun deep towards S 4 (146) or LI
20 (100).

S 4 (146)

Location: 0.4 tsun beside the angle of the mouth.

Indications: Bell's palsy, Salivation, Toothache.

Method of Insertion: Straight insertion of 0.5 − 0.7 tsun
deep or slanting insertion towards
S 6 (148).

S 6 (148)

Location: 0.5 tsun anterior and superior to the angle of the
mandible.

Indications: Toothache, Bell's palsy, Spasm of Masseteric
muscle.

Method of Insertion: Straight or slanting insertion of 0.5
tsun towards the front side.

S 7 (149)

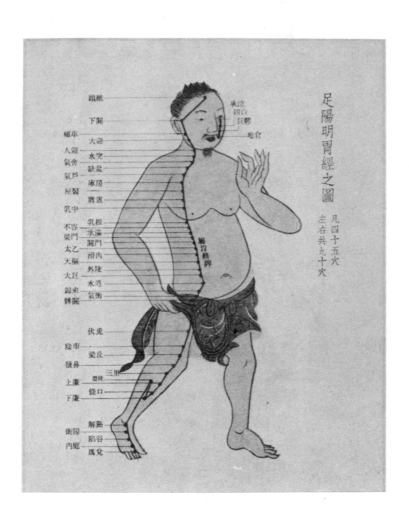

Fig. 10　The Leg Sunlight Yang Stomach Meridian

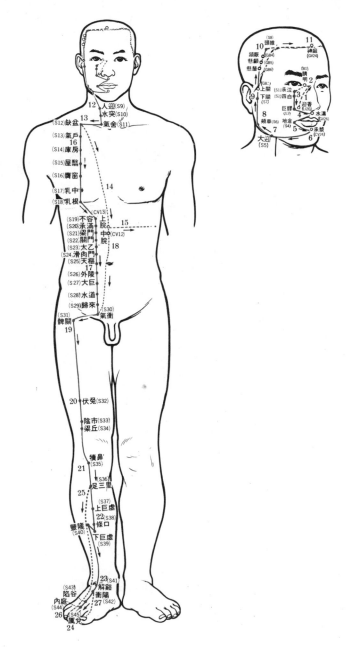

Fig. 11　The Leg Sunlight Yang Stomach Meridian

Location: 1.5 tsun above S 6 (148) at the lower border of
the zygomatic arch.
Indications: Upper molar toothache, Mandibular arthritis.
Method of Insertion: Straight insertion of 0.5 − 1.0 tsun deep.

S 8 (150)
Location: 0.5 tsun above the angle of the forehead hairline.
Indications: Migraine, Giddiness.
Method of Insertion: Horizontal insertion towards GB 14
(201) and about 2 tsun deep.

S 18 (160)
Location: On the nipple line in the fifth intercostal space.
Indications: Poor lactation, Intercostal neuralgia.
Method of Insertion: Slanting insertion of 0.5 − 0.8 tsun
deep.

S 25 (167)
Location: 2 tsun beside the umbilicus.
Indications: Acute or Chronic gastro-enteritis, Appendicitis,
Distension of the abdomen.
Method of Insertion: Stright insertion of 1 − 1.5 tsun deep.

S 34 (176)
Location: 2 tsun above the patella along its lateral border.
Indications: Knee pain, Weakness of knee, Gastric pain.
Method of Insertion: Straight insertion of 1-2 tsun deep

or slanting insertion downwards to the patella.

S 35 (177)

Location: Inferior lateral part of the patella, right over the lateral knee eye.

Indications: Arthritis of knee.

Method of Insertion: Slanting insertion towards the superior medial direction about 0.5 — 1.0 tsun deep.

S 36 (178)

Location: 3 tsun below S 35 (177) or 4 tsun below the middle of patella, 1 tsun beside the anterior border of the tibia.

Indications: Indigestion, Abdominal distension, Gastritis, Vomiting, Hemiplegia, special treatment for upper gastric-intestine tract diseases.

Method of Insertion: Straight insertion of 1 — 1.5 tsun or slanting insertion 1.5 tsun deep.

S40 (182)

Location: 8 tsun above the prominence of the lateral malleolus.

Indications: Cough, Excessive sputum, Vertigo, Paralysis of lower extremities.

Method of Insertion: Straight insertion of 1 — 2 tsun deep.

S 41 (183)

Location: In the middle of the transverse malleolar crease on the dorsal surface of the ankle.

Indications: Drop foot, Hemiplegia.

Method of Insertion: Straight insertion of 0.5 tsun or slanting insertion downward 1 − 2 tsun deep.

S 44 (186)

Location: 0.5 tsun proximal to the web between the second and third toe.

Indications: Toothache, Hemiplegia, Headache.

Method of Insertion: Straight insertion of 0.3 − 0.5 tsun or slanting insertion 0.5 − 1 tsun deep.

Chapter 6

The Leg Greater Yin Spleen
Meridian and points

I. The Leg Greater Yin Spleen Meridian

There are a total of 21 points on this meridian.

(A) Direction:

It starts at the medial side of the nail of the big toe, goes up to the anterior border of the medial malleolus, ascends to the knee, thigh and joins the Conception vessel at CV 3, CV 4 and CV 10. It then runs to the stomach and spleen. (Fig. 12, Fig. 13)

(B) Branches:

The first internal branch: from the stomach goes through the diaphragm to the heart.

The second mixed branch: starts at the CV 10 point, upward to the side of the chest and along the oesophagus ascends to the base of the tongue.

(C) Connected Internal Organs:

Spleen, Stomach, Heart, Lung and Intestine.

(D) Connective points:

CV 3, CV 4, CV 10 (the Conception Vessel)

GB 24 (the Leg Lesser Yang Gall Bladder Meridian)

Liv. 14 (the Leg Absolute Yin Liver Meridian)

L1 (the Arm Greater Yin Lung Meridian)

The termination of this meridian connects with the Arm Lesser Yin Heart Meridian at the heart region.

II Commonly Used Points

SP 1 (299)

Location: 0.1 tsun proximal to the corner of nail on the medial side of the big toe.

Indications: Convulsion, Insanity, Excessive dreaming, Insomnia.

Method of Insertion: Straight insertion of 0.1 − 0.2 tsun deep.

SP 6 (304)

Location: 3 tsun above the prominence of the medial malleolus at the posterior border of tibia.

Indications: Urogenital disease, such as Irregular menstruation, Dysmenorrhoea, Nocturnal emission, Enuresis, Dysuria, Neurasthesia, special treatment for urinary-genital organs diseases of the lady.

Method of Insertion : Straight insertion of 0.5 tsun − 1.5 tsun deep or point to point insertion towards GB 39 (226).

SP 9 (307)

Locations: Below the lower border of the medial condyle

of the tibia, at the level of GB 34 (221).

Indications: Enuresis, Dysuria, Knee pain.

Method of Insertion: Straight insertion of 1.0 − 1.5 tsun
deep or point to point insertion
towards GB 34 (221).

SP 10 (308)

Location: 2 tsun above the superior medial border of the
patella.

Indications: Menorrhagia, thigh pain, special treatment for
dermatologic diseases such as urticaria.

Method of Insertion: Straight or slanting insertion of 1.0 −
1.5 tsun deep.

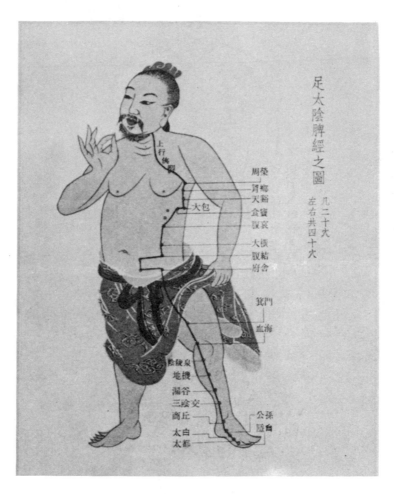

Fig. 12　The Leg Greater Yin Spleen Meridian

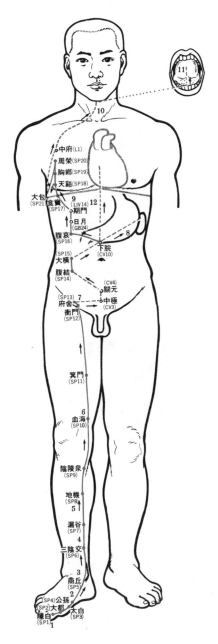

中府(L1)
周榮(SP20)
胸鄉(SP19)
天谿(SP18)
大包(SP21)
食竇(SP17)
9
(LIV14) 12
期門
日月(GB24)
腹哀(SP16)
下脘(CV10)
8
大橫(SP15)
腹結(SP14)
(CV4)
關元
(SP13) 7
府舍
中極(CV3)
衝門(SP12)
箕門(SP11)
血海(SP10) 6
陰陵泉(SP9)
地機(SP8) 5
漏谷(SP7) 4
三陰交(SP6)
商丘(SP5) 3
公孫(SP4) 2
大都(SP2)
隱白(SP1) 1
太白(SP3)
10
11

Fig. 13　The Leg Greater Yin Spleen Meridian

Chapter 7

The Arm Lesser Yin Heart Meridian and points

I. The Arm Lesser Yin Heart Meridian

There are a total of 9 points on this meridian.

(A) Direction:

It starts at the heart, goes around the tissue of the heart, then descends through the diaphragm and connects with the small intestine.

(B) Branches:

The first upper internal branch:from the heart ascends along the oesophagus to the eye.

The second mixed branch: from the heart to lung, joins with the superficial branch at the medial axillary artery, then descends to the ulnar side of the arm and end on the radial side of the tip of the little finger.

(C) Connected Internal Organs:

Heart, Small Intestine, Lung and Kidney.

(D) Connective Points:

None.

The termination of this meridian connects with the Arm Greater Yang Small Intestine Meridian at the tip of the little finger.

II. Commonly Used Points:

H 1 (72)

Location: Middle of the armpit, at the medial side of the axillary artery.

Indications: Angina pictoria, Costalgia.

Method of Insertion: Straight insertion of 0.5 − 1.0 tsun deep.

H 3 (74)

Location: The medial end of the elbow crease when the elbow is flexed.

Indications: Elbow pain.

Method of Insertion: Straight insertion of 0.5 − 1.5 tsun deep.

H 5 (76)

Location: 1 tsun above H 7 (78) on the ulnar side of the forearm.

Indications: Aphasia, Painful wrist.

Method of Insertions: Straight insertion of 0.3 tsun deep.

H 7 (78)

Location: The most distal skin crease of wrist on the ulnar side.

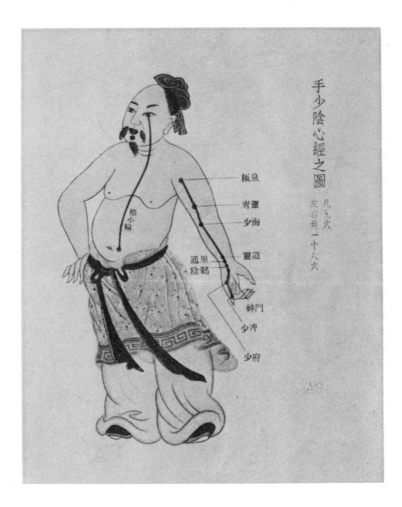

手少陰心經之圖

凡九穴
左右共一十八穴

極泉
青靈
少海
靈道
通里
陰郄
神門
少冲
少府

絡小腸

Fig. 14   The Arm Lesser Yin Heart Meridian

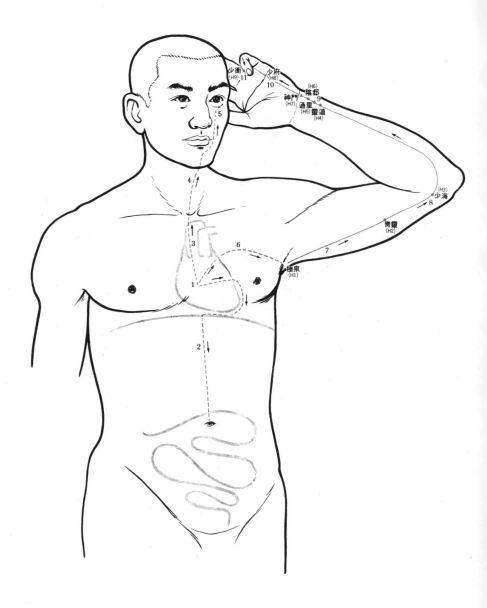

Fig. 15　The Arm Lesser Yin Heart Meridian

Indications: Excessive dreaming, Insomnia, Palpitation, Anxiety, Hysteria.

Method of Insertion: Straight or slanting insertion of 0.5 tsun deep.

H 8 (79)

Location: Between the fourth and fifth metacarpal bones where the tip of the little finger touches on clenching the fist.

Indications: Palpitation, Enuresis.

Method of Insertion: Straight Insertion of 0.3 − 0.5 tsun deep.

H 9 (80)

Location: 0.1 tsun proximal to the corner of nail of little finger on the radial side.

Indications: Palpitation, Chest pain, Apoplexy.

Method of Insertion: Straight insertion of 0.1 tsun deep.

Chapter 8
The Arm Greater Yang Small Intestine Meridian and points

I. The Arm Greater Yang Small Intestine Meridian.

There are a total of 19 points on this meridian.

(A) Direction:

It starts of the tip of the little finger on the ulnar side, goes up to the wrist, elbow and shoulder area at SI 15 point. It then joins with the Governing Vessel at GV 14 point, then turns to the supraclavicular fossa along the oesophagus and heart, through the diaphragm to the stomach and small intestine. (Fig. 16, Fig. 17)

(B) Branches:

The first external branch: starts at the supraclavicular fossa, goes along the side of neck, up to the lateral canthus and the front of the tragus of the ear, then goes into the ear.

The second internal branch: starts directly above the lower border of the mandible goes up to the inner canthus connects with the Bladder Meridian at B 1 point and to the lower border of the zygomatic bone.

(C) Connected Internal Organs:

Small Intestine, Heart and Stomach.

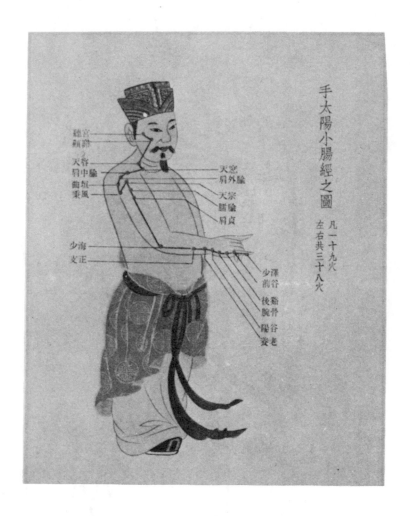

Fig. 16　The Arm Greater Yang Small Intestine Meridian

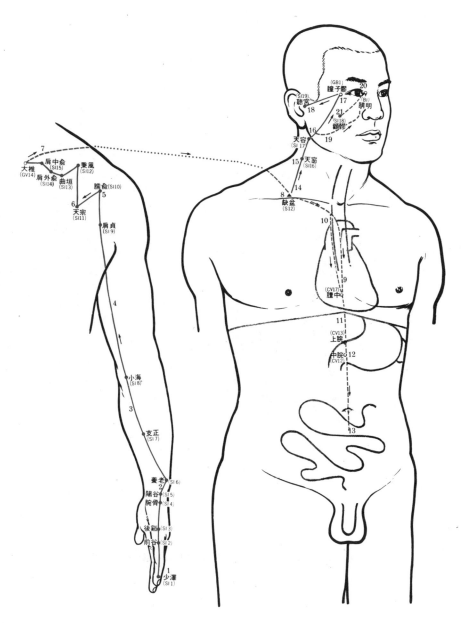

Fig. 17   The Arm Greater Yang Small Intestine Meridian

(D) Connective Points:

GV 14 (The Governing Vessel)

CV 13, CV 12, CV 17 (The Conception Vessel)

B 1 (The Leg Greater Yang Bladder Meridian)

GB 1 (The Leg Lesser Yang Gall-Bladder Meridian)

The termination of this meridian connects with the Leg Greater Yang Bladder Meridian.

II. Commonly Used Points:

SI 1 (124)

Location: 0.1 tsun proximal to the corner of the nail at the ulnar side of the little finger.

Indications: Headache, Poor Lactation.

Method of Insertion: Straight insertion of 0.1 tsun deep.

SI 3 (126)

Location: Ulnar side of the neck of the metacarpal bone of the little finger.

Indications: Intercostal Neuralgia, Lumbago, Night sweating.

Method of Insertion: Straight Insertion of 0.2 tsun or slanting insertion upward 0.5 − 1 tsun deep.

SI 9 (132)

Location: 1 tsun above the posterior axillery fold.

Indications: Shoulder pain, Tinnitus, Deafness.

Method of Insertion: Straight insertion of 1.0 − 1.5 tsun
deep.

SI 12 (135)
Location: Middle of the supra-scapular fossa.
Indications: Scapular pain, Numbness and painful upper arm.
Method of Insertion: Slanting or straight insertion of
1 − 1.5 tsun deep.

SI 18 (141)
Location: On the lower border of the zygomatic bone on
the lateral canthus line.
Indications: Bell's palsy, Toothache.
Method of Insertion: Straight or slanting insertion of 0.5
tsun deep.

SI 19 (142)
Location: Between the middle of the tragus and the man-
dibular joint.
Indications: Deafness, Tinnitus.
Method of Insertion: Straight insertion of 0.5 tsun deep.

Chapter 9

The Leg Greater Yang Bladder
Meridian and points

I.   The Leg Greater Yang Bladder Meridian

There are a total of 67 points on this meridian.

(A) Direction:

It starts at 0.1 tsun above the medial canthus and goes up to the middle of the forehead hair line. It then connects with the Governing Vessel at GV 24 point, goes up to the vertex of head, and descends to the Governing Vessel at GV 17, then passes to the occipital hair line, and divides into two lines at B 10. One is 1.5 tsun lateral to the spine. The other is 3 tsun lateral to the spine. Both these branches go down to the buttocks, hip joints and posterior area of thigh to unite at the center of popliteal fossa. It then passes along the lateral border of the lateral side of the little toe. (Fig. 18, Fig. 19)

(B) Branches:

The first internal branch:starts from the vertex runs to the apex of ear and connects with the Gall-Bladder Meridian at GB 8 point. This branch has no points.

The second internal branch: at the B23 point divides an

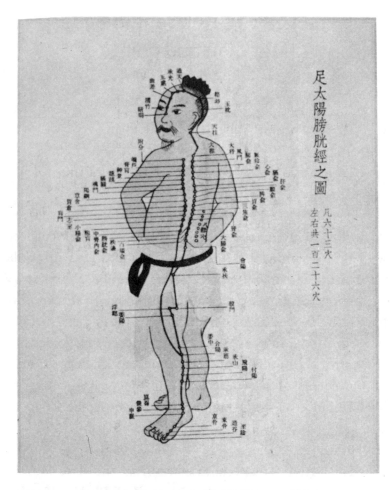

Fig. 18   The Greater Yang Bladder Meridian

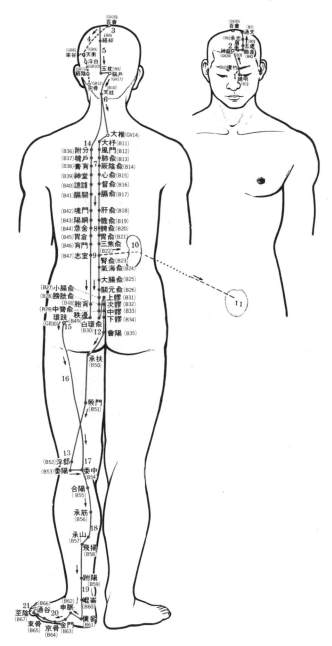

Fig. 19　The Leg Greater Yang Bladder Meridian

inner branch goes to the kidney and Bladder.

(C) Connected Internal Organs:.
Bladder, Kidney, Brain and Heart.

(D) Connective points:
GB 8, GB 9, GB 10, GB 11, GB 12, GB 30 (The Leg Lesser Yang Gall Bladder Meridian)
GV 24, GV 20, GV 17, GV 14 (The Governing Vessel)
The termination of this meridian connects with the Leg Lesser Yin Kidney Meridian at the little toe.

II. Commonly Used Points

B1 (232)
Location: 0.1 tsun above the medial canthus, near the margin of the orbit.
Indications: Myopia, Hypermetropia, Acute Conjunctivitis.
Method of Insertion: Straight insertion of 0.2 − 0.3 tsun deep.

B 2 (233)
Location: At the medial end of the eyebrow.
Indications: Headache, Blurred vision, Bell's Palsy.
Method of Insertion: Straight or slanting insertion of 0.2 − 0.3 tsun deep.

B 10 (241)
Location: Same level as GV 15, on the lateral of the margin

of the trapezius muscle.

Indications: Stiff neck, Neurasthenia, Hysteria, Occipital Headache.

Method of Insertion: Straight insertion of 1.0 – 1.5 tsun deep.

B 12 (243)

Location: 1.5 tsun lateral to the space spinous processes of the second and third thoracic vertebra.

Indications: Common cold, Bronchitis.

Method of Insertion: Straight or slanting insertion of 0.5 – 1.0 tsun deep.

B 13 (244) (Lung locus)

Location: 1.5 tsun lateral to the space spinous process of the third and fourth thoracic vertebra.

Indications: Asthma, Pneumonia, Cough.

Method of Insertion: Straight insertion of 0.5 – 1.0 tsun deep.

B 15 (246) (Heart locus)

Location: 1.5 tsun lateral to the space spinous process of the fifty and sixth thoracic vertebra.

Indications: Palpitation, Hysteria, Schizophrenia.

Method of Insertion: Straight or slanting insertion of 0.5 – 1.0 tsun deep.

B 17 (248) (Diaphragm locus)

Location: 1.5 tsun lateral to the space spinous process of the seventh and eight thoracic vertebra.

Indications: Hiccough, Vomiting, Nausea.

Method of Insertion: Straight or slanting insertion of 0.5 – 1.0 tsun deep.

B 21 (252) (Stomach locus)

Location: 1.5 tsun lateral to the space spinous process of the twelth thoracic vertebra and the first lumbar vertebra.

Indications: Gactric ulcer, Indigestion, Gastroptosis.

Method of Insertion: Slanting or straight insertion of 0.5 – 1.0 tsun deep.

B 23 (254) (Kidney locus)

Location: 1.5 tsun lateral to the space spinous process of the second and third lumbar vertebra.

Indications: Lumbago, Impotence, Noctural emission.

Method of Insertion: Straight insertion of 1.0 – 1.5 tsun deep.

B 25 (256) (Large intestine locus)

Location: 1.5 tsun lateral to the space spinous process of the fourth and fifth lumbar vertebra.

Indications: Constipation, Lumbago, Diarrhoea.

Method of Insertion: Straight insertion of 1.0 – 1.5 tsun deep.

B 31, B 32, B 33, B 34 (262) (263) (264) (265)

Location: In the first, second, third and fourth posterior sacral foramen.

Indications: Dysuria, Enuresis, Sciatica, Irregular menstruation, Neurasthenia.

Method of Insertion: Straight insertion 0.5 – 1.0 tsun deep.

B 47 (or B 52) (278)

Location: 3 tsun lateral to the space spinous process of the second and third lumbar vertebra.

Indications: Lumbago, Impotence, Dysuria.

Method of Insertion: Straight insertion of 1.0 – 1.5 tsun deep.

B 50 (or B 36) (281)

Location: Midpoint of the gluteal fold.

Indications: Sciatica, Paralysis of the lower extremities.

Method of Insertion: Straight insertion of 2 – 3 tsun deep.

B 51 (or B 37) (282)

Location: In the center of the back of the thigh.

Indications: Sciatica, Hemiplegia.

Method of Insertion: Straight insertion of 2–3 tsun deep.

B 54 (or B 40) (285)

Location: Midpoint of the transverse popliteal crease.

Indications: Sciatica, Hemiplegia.

Method of Insertion: Straight insertion of 1 tsun deep.

B 57 (288)

Location: Directly in the apex of the mid point of the lower border of the gastrocnemius muscle.

Indications: Gastrocnemius muscle cramp, Leg pain.

Method of Insertion: Straight insertion of 1.0 — 1.5 tsun deep.

B 60 (291)

Location: Between the posterior border of the lateral malleolus and the tendon achilles, at the same level as K 3 (336).

Indications: Sciatica, Hemiplegia.

Method of Insertion: Straight insertion of 1.0 — 1.5 tsun deep, or point to point towards K 3 (336).

B 67 (298)

Location: 0.1 tsun proximal to the corner of the nail of the little toe on the lateral side.

Indications: Difficult labour.

Method of Insertion: Straight insertion of 0.1 tsun deep.

Chapter 10

The Leg Lesser Yin Kidney Meridian and points

I. The Leg Lesser Yin Kidney Meridian

There are a total of 27 points on this meridian.

(A) Direction:

It originates from the tip of the little toe, becoming superficial in the midline of the junction of the anterior and middle one third part of the plantar surface of the foot. It then goes up to the medial malleolus, along the medial side of thigh and connects with the Governing Vessel at GV 1 point. It then passes along the front of the vetebral column to the kidney and bladder and joins the conception vessel at CV 4 and CV 3, along the side of chest upwards to the first intercostal space. (Fig. 20, Fig. 21)

(B) Branches:

The first internal branch: starts from the kidney, goes upward through the liver, diaphragm, heart, pericardium and lung then goes along the larynx to the base of tongue.

The second internal branch: from the lung runs to the front of trunk at CV 17 point.

(C) Connected Internal Organs:

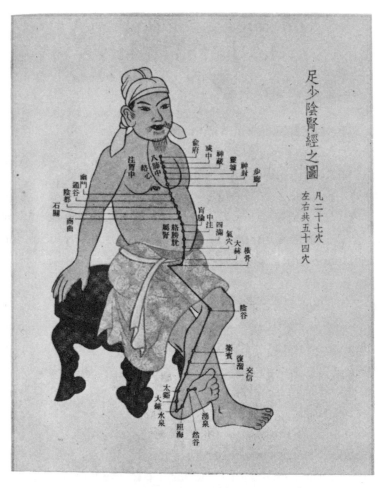

Fig. 20   The Leg Lesser Yin Kidney Meridian

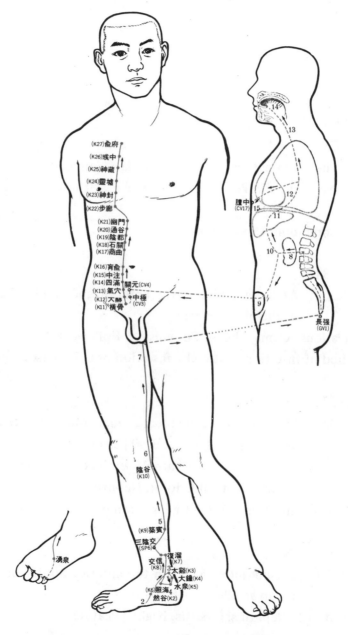

Fig. 21   The Leg Lesser Yin Kidney Meridian

Kidney, Bladder, Liver, Lung, Heart, Pericardium.
(D) Connective Points:
SP 6 (The Leg Great Yin Spleen Meridian)
GV 1 (The Governing Vessel)
CV 3, CV 4 (The Conception Vessel)
The termination of this meridian connects with the Arm Absolute Yin Pericardium Meridian at the pericardium.

II. Commonly Used Points

K 1 (334)
Location: At the junction of the anterior and middle thirds of the plantar area.
Indications: Coma, Shock, Convulsion, Epilepsy.
Method of Insertion: Straight insertion of 0.5 – 1 tsun deep.

K 3 (336)
Location: Midway between medial malleolus and tendo achilles, same level as B 60 (291).
Indications: Enuresis, Nocturnal emission, Impotence, Oedema of ankle joint, Nephritis.
Method of Insertion: Straight insertion of 0.5 – 1 tsun deep.

K 7 (340)
Location: 2 tsun above K 3, on the anterior border of the tendo achilles.
Indications: Nephritis, Cystitis, Night sweating.

Method of Insertion: Straight insertion of 1 — 1.5 tsun deep.

K 16 (349)
Location: 0.5 tsun beside the umbilicus.
Indications: Constipation, Distension of Abdomen, Intestinal
              spasm.
Method of Insertion: Straight insertion of 1 — 1.5 tsun deep.

Chapter 11

The Arm Absolute Yin Pericardium Meridian and points

I. The Arm Absolute Yin Pericardium Meridian

There are a total of 9 points on this meridian.

(A) Direction:

It originates from the upper warmer and pericardium and then descends to the middle and lower warmer. (Fig. 22, Fig. 23)

(B) Branches:

The first mixed branch: starts from the upper warmer to the outer part of the chest and goes upward to the axillary area along the midline of the upper extremities. It then goes down to the palm and ends at the radial side of the tip of the middle finger.

The second internal branch: starts from P 8 and descends to the ulnar side of the ring finger.

(C) Connected Internal Organs:

Pericardium, Triple Warmer.

(D) Connective Points:

CV 17, CV 12, CV 7 (The Conception Vessel Meridian)

The termination of this meridian connects with the Arm Lesser Yang Triple Warmer Meridian at the ulnar side of the ring finger.

II. Commonly Used Points:

P 3 (65)
Location: Middle of the elbow crease, at the ulnar side of the tendon of the biceps brachii muscle.
Indications: Elbow and Arm pain, Palpitation, Fever.
Method of Insertion: Straight insertion of $0.5 - 1$ tsun deep.

P 5 (67)
Location: 3 tsun above P 7 (69) at the midline of the ventral surface of the arm.
Indications: Vomiting, Fever, Asthma, Schizophrenia.
Method of Insertion: Straight insertion of $0.5 - 1$ tsun deep.

P 6 (68)
Location: 2 tsun above P 7 (69)
Indications: Hiccough, Vomiting, Nausea, Hysteria, insomnia, special treatment for thoracic organs diseases.
Method of Insertion: Straight insertion of $0.5 - 1$ tsun deep or point to point toward T 5 (105).

P 7 (69)
Location: Middle of the most distal skin crease of wrist.
Indications: Painful wrist and its surrounding soft tissue.

Method of Insertion: Straight insertion of 0.3 – 0.5 tsun
deep.

P 8 (70)

Location: Between the second and third metacarpal bone
where the tip of the middle finger touches when
the fist is clenched.

Indications: Convulsion, Hiccough, Insanity.

Method of Insertion: Straight insertion of 0.3 – 0.5 tsun
deep.

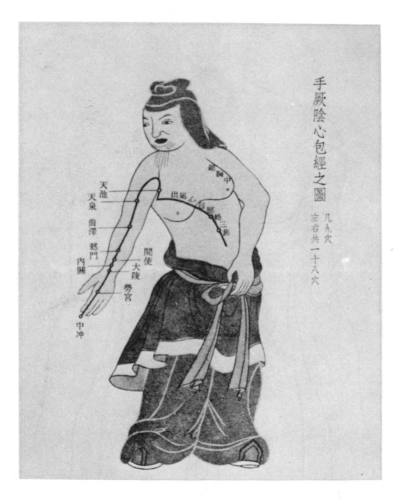

Fig. 22　The Arm Absolute Yin Pericardium Meridian

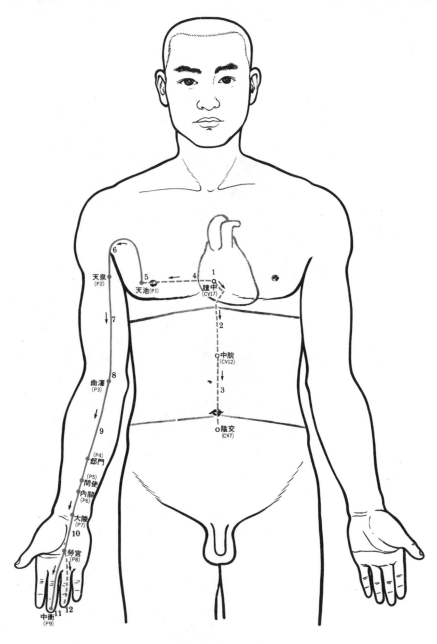

天泉 (P2)

天池(P1)

膻中 (CV17)

中脘 (CV12)

陰交 (CV7)

曲澤 (P3)

(P4) 郄門

(P5) 間使

內關 (P6)

大陵 (P7)

勞宮 (P8)

中衝 (P9)

Fig. 23   The Arm Absolute Yin Pericardium Meridian

Chapter 12
The Arm Lesser Yang Triple Warmer Meridian and points

I. **The Arm Lesser Yang Triple Warmer Meridian**

There are a total of 23 points on this meridian.

(A) Direction:

It originates from the ulna side of the tip of the ring finger, goes upwards to the web of the ring finger and the little finger, then up the forearm and connects with the Leg Lesser Yang Gall Bladder Meridian at GB 21. It then goes into the supraclavicular fossa and runs down to the pericardium, diaphragm and upper, middle and lower warmer. (Fig. 24, Fig. 25)

(B) Branches:

The first mixed branch: starts at the level of the fourth intercostal space between the nipples at CV 17, goes up to supraclavicular fossa, neck and mastoid, twists around the posterior border of the auricular area and reaches the zygomatic bone and joins the Arm Greater Yang Small Intestine Meridian at SI 18.

The second external branch: starts at T 17, runs into the

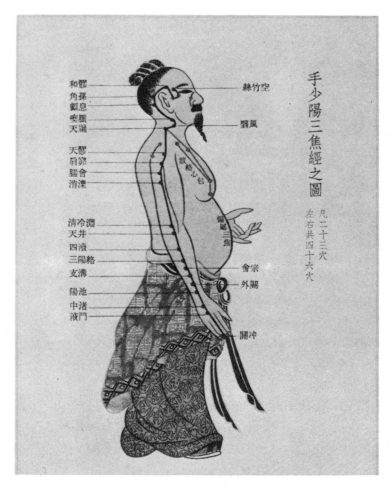

Fig. 24　The Arm Lesser Yang Triple Warmer Meridian

70

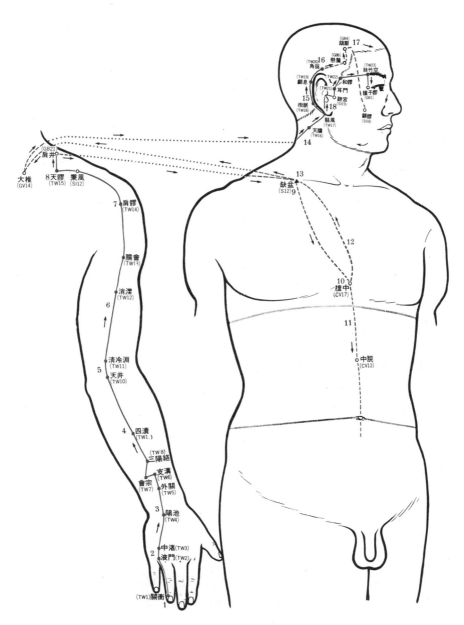

Fig. 25　The Arm Lesser Yang Triple Warmer Meridian

ear and goes along the anterior border of auricular area. Then goes up to the lateral canthus, and connects with the Leg Lesser Yang Gall Bladder Meridian at GB 1.

(C) Connected Internal Organs:

Triple Warmer, Pericardium.

(D) Connective Points:

SI 12, SI 18, SI 19 (The Arm Greater Yang Small Intestine Meridian)

GB 1, GB 4, GB 6, GB 21 (The Leg Lesser Yang Gall Bladder Meridian)

GV 14 (Governing Vessel)

CV 17, CV 12 (The Conception Vessel Meridian)

The termination of this meridian connects with the Leg Lesser Yang Gall Bladder Meridian.

II. Commonly Used Points

T 2 (102)

Location: 0.5 tsun proximal to the web between the ring and the small fingers.

Indications: Headache, Deafness, Ring finger pain.

Method of Insertion: Straight Insertion of 0.3 − 0.5 tsun deep.

T 3 (103)

Location: 1 tsun proximal to point T 2 (102)

Indications: Tinnitus, Numbness of ring finger.

Method of Insertion: Straight insertion of 0.5 tsun deep.

T 5 (105)

Location: 2 tsun proximal to the skin crease of dorsum of wrist.

Indications: Hemiplegia, Deafness, Tinnitus, Fever.

Method of Insertion: Straight or slanting insertion of 0.5 – 1 tsun deep.

T 10 (110)

Location: 1 tsun proximal to the olecranon when the elbow is slightly flexed.

Indications: Elbow pain.

Method of Insertion: Straight insertion of 0.5 – 1 tsun deep.

T 14 (114)

Location: At the postero-inferior part of the acromion, same level as LI 15 (95).

Indications: Shoulder pain, Frozen shoulder.

Method of Insertion: Slanting insertion of 0.5 – 1 tsun deep.

T 17 (117)

Location: Posterior to the lobe of ear, between the angle of mandible and the mastoid process.

Indications: Deafness, Tinnitus, Bell's palsy.

Method of Insertion: Slanting insertion of 1.0 – 1.5 tsun deep.

T 21 (121)

Location: The front of the upper part of the tragus, above the SI 19 (142).

Indications: Deafness, Tinnitus, Toothache.

Method of Insertion: Straight or slanting insertion of 0.5 – 1 tsun downwards.

T 23 (123)

Location: Lateral end of the eyebrow.

Indications: Migraine, Headache.

Method of insertion: Slanting or horizontal insertion of 0.5 tsun deep.

Chapter 13

The Leg Lesser Yang Gall Bladder Meridian and points

I. The Leg Lesser Yang Gall Bladder Meridian

There are a total of 44 points on this meridian.

(A) Direction:

It starts at the lateral canthus, goes to the tragus of the ear and the temporal area. It curves back and forth on the side of the head, then goes to the back of neck, connects with the Governing Vessel at GV 14, runs back to the supraclavicular fossa and runs down to the axillary area, the lateral side of the chest and the abdomen connects with the Leg Greater Yang Bladder Meridian at B 31 and B 32. It then runs along the lateral side of the thigh and leg to the fourth toe. (Fig. 26, Fig. 27)

(B) Branches:

The first internal branch: starts from the lateral canthus, goes downwards and joins the Arm Greater Yang Small Intestine Meridian at SI 18. It then runs down to the supraclavicular fossa and passes through the diaphragm to the liver and gallbladder, meeting the main branch (direction) at the

GB 30 point.

The second internal branch: starts at GB 41 point, divides into a small inner branch and runs to the tip of the big toe.

(C) Connected Internal Organs:

Gallbladder, Liver, Heart.

(D) Connective points:

T 17, T 20, T 22 (the Arm Lesser Yang Triple Warmer Meridian).

SI 18, SI 19, SI 12 (the Arm Greater Yang Small Intestine Meridian).

GV 14 (Governing Vessel)

Liv 13 (the Leg Absolute Yin Liver Meridian).

The termination of this meridian connects with the Leg Absolute Yin Liver Meridian at the distal phalanx of the big toe.

II.   Commonly Used Points:

GB 1 (188)

Location: 0.5 tsun lateral to the external cathus.

Indications: Optic nerve atrophy, Keratitis.

Method of Insertion: Slanting insertion of 0.2 − 0.3 tsun deep.

GB 2 (189)

Location: 0.5 tsun below SI 19 (142), anterior to the tragic

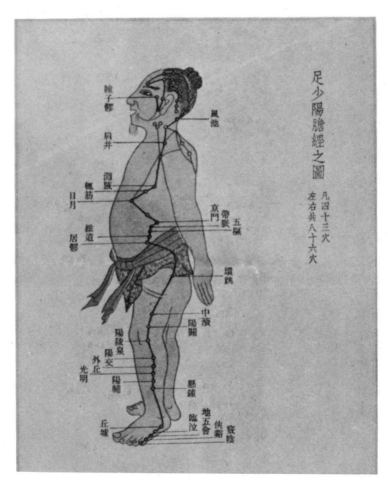

瞳子髎
肩井
淵腋
輒筋
日月
維道
居髎

風池
京門
帶脈
五樞
環跳
中瀆
陽關
陽陵泉
陽交
外丘
光明
陽輔
懸鍾
丘墟
臨泣
地五會
俠谿
竅陰

足少陽膽經之圖 凡四十三穴 左右共八十六穴

Fig. 26   The Leg Lesser Yang Gall-Bladder Meridian

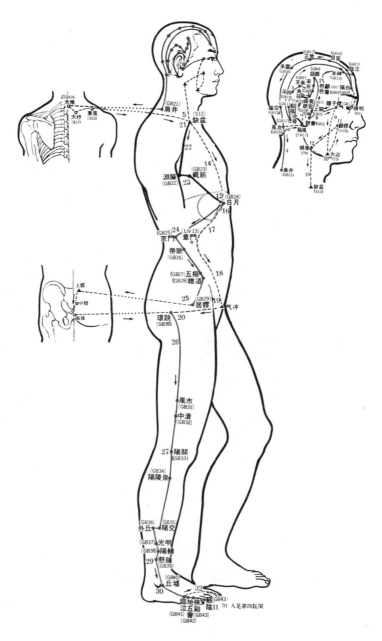

Fig. 27　The Leg Lesser Yang Gall-Bladder Meridian

notch.

Indications: Deafness, Tinnitus.

Method of Insertion: Straight insertion of 0.3 – 0.5 tsun deep.

GB 3 (190)

Location: At the front of the ear on the upper border of the zygomatic arch.

Indications: Toothache, Bell's palsy.

Method of Insertion: Straight or slanting insertion of 0.5 tsun deep.

GB 8 (195)

Location: 1.5 tsun above apex of ear.

Indications: Migraine, Vertigo, Amnesia.

Method of Insertion: Slanting or horizontal insertion of 1 – 1.5 tsun deep.

GB 14 (201)

Location: 1 tsun above the middle of the eyebrow.

Indications: Bell's palsy, Headache, Trigeminal neuralgia.

Method of Insertion: Slanting insertion or horizontal insertion of 0.3 – 0.5 tsun deep.

GB 20 (207)

Location: At the lateral border of trapezuis muscle, 1 tsun above the occipital hairline, same level as GV 16

(12).

Indications: Common cold, Fever, Wry neck, occipital area pain, Hypertension.

Method of Insertion: Straight insertion of 1.0 − 1.5 tsun or slanting insertion of 1.5 tsun downward.

GB 21 (208)

Location: Midway between GV 14 (14) and the acromion.

Indications: Shoulder pain, Wry neck.

Method of Insertion: Straight insertion of 1.0 − 1.5 tsun deep.

GB 30 (217)

Location: one-third distance from the greater, great trochanter of the femur to the hiatus of the sacrum.

Indications: Sciatica, Hemiplegia, Lumbago.

Method of Insertion: Straight insertion of 1.5 − 3.0 tsun deep.

GB 34 (221)

Location: 2 tsun below the middle of patella at the lateral line of the leg.

Indications: Cholecystitis, Hemiplegia, special treatment for liver, gall-bladder diseases.

Method of Insertion: Straight insertion of 1.0 − 1.5 tsun deep.

GB 37 (224) (Bright Point)

Location: 5 tsun above the prominence of the lateral malleolus.

Indications: Blurred vision, Night blindness.

Method of Insertion: Straight insertion of 1.0 tsun deep.

GB 39 (226)

Location: 3 tsun above the prominence of the lateral malleolus.

Indications: Ankle joint pain, Hemiplegia, sciatica.

Method of Insertion: Straight insertion of 0.5 − 1.0 tsun deep or point to point towards SP 6. (304).

Chapter 14
The Leg Absolute Yin Liver Meridian and points

I. The Leg Absolute Yin Liver Meridian

There are a total of 14 points on this meridian.

It originates from the lateral side of the distal phalanx of the big toe, goes up to the front of the medial malleolus, connects with the Leg Greater Yin Spleen Meridian at SP 6 point, then runs past the spleen meridian, goes along the medial side of leg and turns at the external genital organs. It then goes to the lateral side of abdomen, connects with the liver, gallbladder, stomach and kidney, passes through the diaphragm, runs along the posterior border of the trachea, then goes upward to the eye, forehead and joins the governing vessel at the vertex. (Fig. 28 , Fig 29)

(B) Branches:

The first internal branch — starts below the eye, then goes down to the angle of mouth and around the lips.

The second internal branch — starts from the liver, passes through the diaphragm to the lung.

(C) Connected Internal Organs:

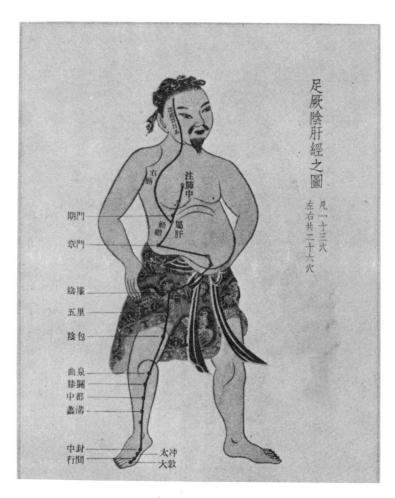

Fig. 28　The Leg Absolute Yin Liver Meridian

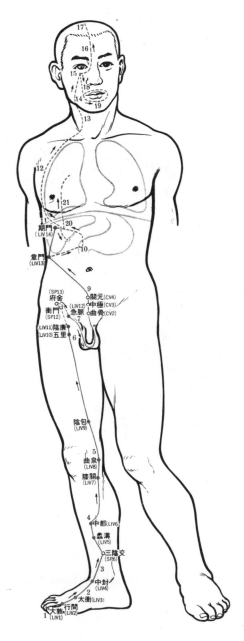

Fig. 29　The Leg Absolute Yin Liver Meridian

Liver, Gallbladder, Lung, Stomach, Kidney, Brain.

(D) Connective Points:

SP 6, SP 12, SP 13 (the Leg Greater Yin Spleen Meridian)

CV 2, CV 3, CV 4 (Conception Vessel)

The termination of this meridian connects with the Arm Greater Yin Lung Meridian at the lung region.

II. Commonly Used Points:

Liv 2 (321)

Location: 0.5 tsun proximal end of the web between the big toe and the second toe.

Indications: Headache, Night Sweating.

Method of Insertion: Straight or slanting insertion upward 0.3 – 0.5 tsun.

Liv 3 (322)

Location: 1.5 tsun proximal to Liv 2 (321).

Indications: Dizziness, Epilepsy, Headache.

Method of Insertion: Slanting insertion, upward, 0.5 tsun.

Liv 8 (327)

Location: Medial end of the knee crease.

Indications: Arthritis of the knee.

Method of Insertion: Straight insertion of 1.0 – 1.5 tsun deep.

Liv 13 (332)

Location: At the end of the eleventh rib, on the anterior axillary line.

Indications: Intercostal neuralgia, Hepatitis, Vomiting.

Method of Insertion: Slanting insertion of 0.5 − 1.0 tsun deep.

Liv 14 (333)

Location: At the sixth intercostal space, on the mammillary line.

Indications: Hepatitis, Intercostal Neuralgia.

Method of Insertion: Slanting insertion of 0.5 − 1.0 tsun deep.

Chapter 15
The Governing Vessel and points

I. The Governing Vessel

There are a total of 28 points on this meridian.

(A) Direction:

It orginates between the tip of the coccyx and the anus, then goes up to the midline of the sacrum, the back and neck, at the 1 tsun above the occipital hairline it runs into the brain and passes GV 16 point to go up to the vertex of head, then goes down to the forehead, nose, and the end at the mid point between the inner surface of the upper lip and the gum. (Fig. 30, Fig. 31)

(B) Branches:

The first internal branch: Starts from the coccyx, goes downward to the perineum and connects with the conception vessel at CV 1.

The second internal branch: Starts between the third and fourth thoracic vertebra and runs to join the Leg Greater Yang Bladder Meridian at B 12 point.

(C) Connected Internal Organs:

Kidney, Brain, Heart, etc.

(D) Connective points:
B 12 (the Leg Greater Yang Bladder Meridian)
CV 1 (the Conception Vessel)

II. Commonly Used Points:

GV 1 (27)
Location: In between the tip of the coccyx and the anus.
Indications: Hemorrhoids, Painful coccyx.
Method of Insertion: Slanting insertion 1.0 − 1.5 tsun deep.

GV 4 (24)
Location: Between the second and the third lumbar vertebra,
           at the midline of the back.
Indications: Lumbago, Impotence, Enuresis, Endometritis.
Method of Insertion: Slanting insertion of 0.5 − 1.0 tsun
                       deep.

GV 14 (14)
Location: Between the seventh cervical vertebra and the
           first thoracic vertebra.
Indications: Fever, Schizophrenia, Asthma, Back pain,
             stiff neck.
Method of Insertion: Slanting insertion of 0.5 − 1.0 tsun
                       deep.

GV 15 (13)

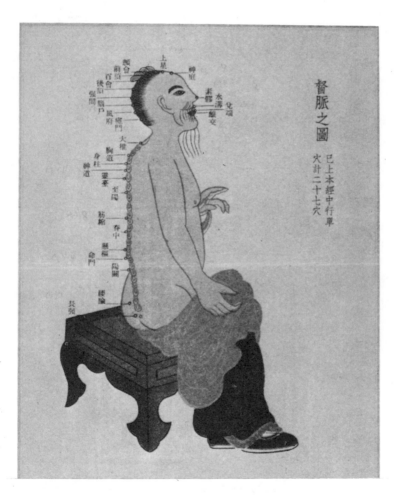

Fig. 30　The Governing Vessel Meridian

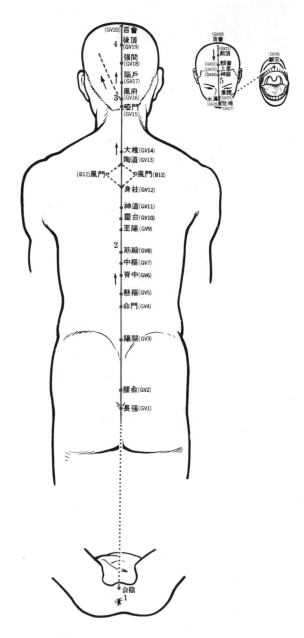

Fig. 31　The Governing Vessel Meridian

Location: 0.5 tsun above occipital hairline, between the first and the second cervical vertebra.

Indications: Deafness, Posterior headache, Insanity.

Method of Insertion: Straight insertion or slanting insertion of 1.0 tsun downward.

GV 16 (12)

Location: 1 tsun above GV 15 (13) point, below the occipital protuberance.

Indications: Apoplexy, Headache, Stiff neck.

Method of Insertion: Straight insertion of 0.5 − 1.0 tsun deep.

GV 20 (8)

Location: 5 tsun posterior to the middle of the natural forehead hairline, mid-way between the apex of both ears.

Indications: Magraine, Vertigo, Neurasthenia, Amnesia.

Method of Insertion: Slanting or Horizontal insertion of 0.5 − 1.0 tsun deep.

GV 24 (4)

Location: Middle of the forehead hairline.

Indications: Vertigo, Dizziness, Insomnia, Frontal headache.

Method of Insertion: Slanting insertion of 0.5 − 1 tsun deep.

GV 26 (2)

Location: Upper one-third point of the philtrum.

Indications: Shock,   Collapse,   Coma,   Hysteria,   Epilepsy.

Method of Insertion: Straight or slanting insertion of 0.3
tsun upward.

GV 27 (1)

Location: The junction of philtrum and upper lip.

Indications: Toothache.

Method of insertion: Slanting or straight insertion of 0.2
— 0.3 tsun deep.

Chapter 16
The Conception Vessel and points

I. The Conception Vessel

There are a total of 24 points on this meridian.

(A) Direction:

It originates from the pubic symphysis, runs to the anterior midline of the abdomen, chest and throat, then around the mouth and goes upwards to the eye. (Fig. 32, Fig. 33)

(B) Branch:

The first internal branch: starts from the public symphysis and runs to the perineum.

The second internal branch: starts from the middle of the mentolabial sulcus and connects with the Governing Vessel at GV 28 point.

(C) Connected Internal Organs:

None

(D) Connective points:

S 1 (The Leg Sunlight Yang Stomach Meridian)

GV 28 (The Governing Vessel)

II. Commonly Used points:

CV 2 (50)

Location: At the upper border of the public symphysis.

Indications: Impotence, Irregular menstruation, Enuresis, Nocturnal emission.

Method of Insertion: Straight insertion of 0.5 − 1.0 tsun deep.

CV 4 (48)

Location: 3 tsun below the umbilicus.

Indications: Dysmenorrhoea, Impotence, Diarrhoea.

Method of Insertion: Straight or slanting insertion of 1.0 − 1.5 tsun deep.

CV 6 (46)

Location: 1.5 tsun below the umbilicus.

Indications: Abdominal distention, Neurasthenia, Enuresis.

Method of Insertion: Straight insertion of 1 − 1.5 tsun deep.

CV 8 (44)

Location: At the center of the umbilicus.

Indications: Diarrhoea, Abdominal pain.

Method of Insertion: Moxibustion only, needling should be avoided.

CV 10 (42)

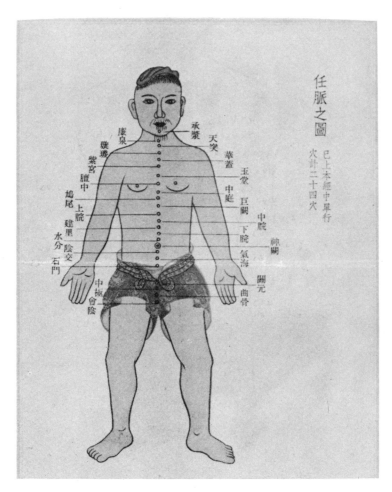

Fig. 32 The Conception Vessel Meridian

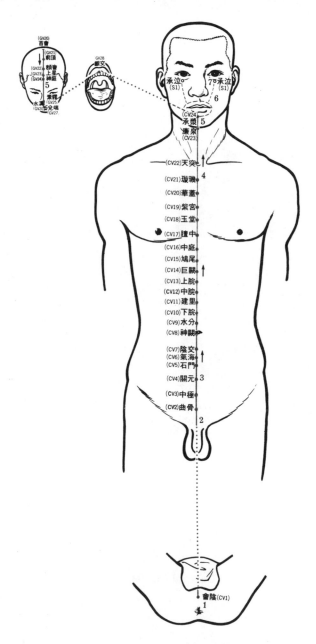

Fig. 33   The Conception Vessel Meridian

Location: 2 tsun above the umbilicus.

Indications: Indigestion, Gastroptosis, Enteritis.

Method of Insertion: Straight insertion of 1.0 − 1.5 tsun deep.

CV 12 (40)

Location: 4 tsun above the umbilicus, middle of the xyphoid process and umbilicus.

Indications: Gastroptosis, Vomiting, Gastric ulcer.

Method of Insertion: Straight insertion of 1 − 2 tsun deep.

CV 13 (39)

Location: 5 tsun above the umbilicus.

Indications: Hiccough, Vomiting, Gastric ulcer.

Method of Insertion: Straight insertion of 1 − 2 tsun deep.

CV 17 (35)

Location: Same level as the fourth intercostal space, at the midline in front of the trunk.

Indications: Hiccough, Bronchial asthma, Bronchitis, Poor lactation.

Method of Insertion: Slanting or horizontal insertion of 0.5 − 1 tsun deep.

CV 22 (30)

Location: Middle of the suprasternal notch.

Indications: Asthma, Bronchitis, vomiting and hiccough.

Method of Insertion: Horizontal insertion along side the trachea 1.0 — 1.5 tsun deep.

CV 23 (29)

Location: Middle of the upper border of the hyoid bone.

Indications: Aphasia, Laryngopharyngitis, Deaf-mutes.

Method of Insertion: Slanting insertion of 0.5 — 1.0 tsun towards the root of the tongue.

CV 24 (28)

Location: At the middle of the mento-labial sulcus.

Indications: Bell's palsy, Toothache, Salivation, Trismus.

Method of Insertion: Straight or slanting insertion of 0.3 — 0.5 tsun deep.

Chapter 17
Chong Mai

(A) Direction:

Originates in the pelvic cavity, runs along the Leg Lesses Yin Kidney Meridian up to the thorax and goes to the upper lip. (Fig. 34)

(B) Branch:

The internal branch — descends to the perineum, pass through the CV 1 then runs up to the vetebral column.

(C) Connected Internal Organ:

None.

(D) Connective points:

CV 1 (The Conception Vessel)

K 11 — K 21 (The Leg Lesser Yin Kidney Meridian)

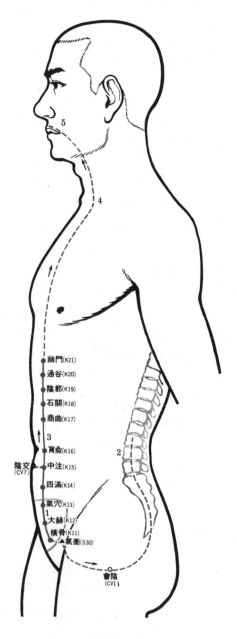

幽門(K21)
通谷(K20)
隆都(K19)
石關(K18)
商曲(K17)
3
肓兪(K16)
陰交 中注(K15)
(CV7)
四滿(K14)
氣穴(K13)
1
大赫(K12)
橫骨(K11)
氣衝(S30)
會陰
(CV1)

Fig. 34 Chong Mai

Chapter 18
Dai Mai (The Belt channel)

(A) Direction:

Originates below the hypochondrium, on the same level as the second lumbar vertebra, runs down along the lateral side of loin and connects with GB 26, GB 27, GB 28, just like a belt. (Fig. 35)

(B) Branches:

None

(C) Connected Internal Organs:

None

(D) Connective Points:

GB 26, GB 27, GB 28 (The Leg Lesser Yang Gall Bladder Meridian)

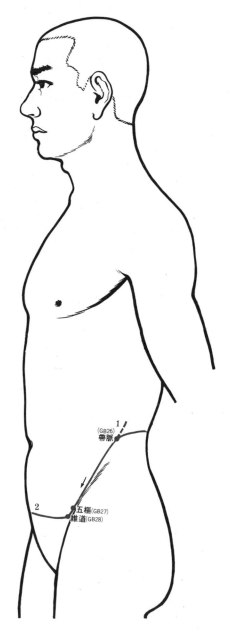

Fig. 35 Dai Mai

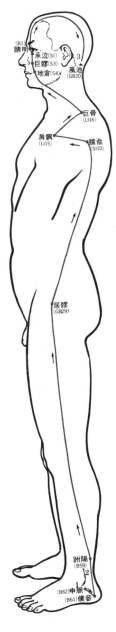

Fig. 36 Yang Chiao Mai

Chapter 19

Yang Chiao Mai

(The Yang motility channel)

(A) Direction:

Originates below the lateral malleolus, ascends along the lateral side of the leg and thigh, then goes up to the shoulder along the side of neck to the angle of mouth. It runs upwards to the inner canthus, and connects with the Yin Chiao Mai through the forehead hairline to the back of head at GB 20. (Fig. 36)

(B) Branches:

None

(C) Connected Internal Organs:

None

(D) Connective Points:

B 62, B 61, B 59, B 1 (the Leg Greater Yang Bladder Meridian)

GB 29, GB 20, (the Leg Lesser Yang Gall-bladder Meridian)

SI 10 (the Arm Greater Yang Small Intestine Meridian)

LI 15, LI 16 (the Arm Sunlight Yang Large Intestine Meridian)

S 4, S 3, S 1 (the Leg Sunlight Yang Stomach Meridian)

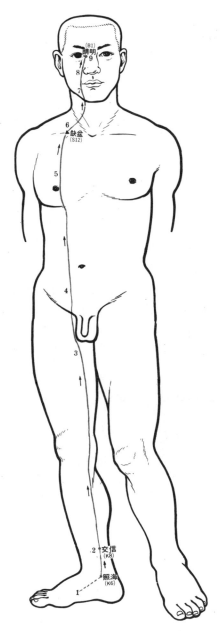

Fig. 37   Yin Chaio Mei

Chapter 20
Yin Chiao Mai
(The Yin motility channel)

(A) Direction:

Originates on the posterior side of the navicular bone, then runs to the medial malleolus, goes upwards along the medial side of leg and thigh, to the external genital organs, then upwards to the supraclavicular fossa, and along the throat to the medial canthus until it joins the Yang Chiao Mai and runs with it to the brain. (Fig. 37)

(B) Branches:

None

(C) Connected Internal Organs:

None

(D) Connective Points:

K 6, K 8 (the Leg Lesser Yin Kidney Meridian)

B 1 (the Leg Greater Yang Bladder Meridian)

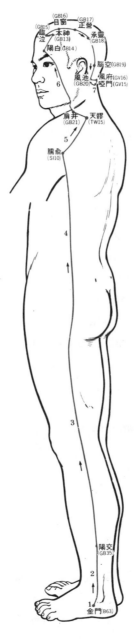

Fig. 38　Yang Wai Mai

Chapter 21
Yang Wai Mai
(The Yang regulation channel)

(A) Direction:

Originates from the Leg Greater Yang Bladder Meridian at point B 63, runs along the lateral side of the leg, and thigh, to the hip and further up to the side of the abdomen and chest. It then runs to the shoulder and neck whence it goes up to the side of the head, then turns backward to the head and connects with the Leg Lesser Yang Gall Bladder Meridian at GB 20 and the Governing Vessel at GV 16, GV 15. (Fig. 38)

(B) Branches:

None

(C) Connected Internal Organs:

None

(D) Connective Points:

B 63 (the Leg Greater Yang Bladder Meridian)

GB 13, GB 14, GB 15, GB 16, GB 17, GB 18, GB 19, GB 20, GB 21, GB 35 (the Leg Lesser Yang Gall-Bladder Meridian)

GV 16, GV 15 (the Governing Vessel Meridian)

SI 10 (the Arm Greater Yang Small Intestine Meridian)

T 15 (the Arm Lesser Yang Triple Warmer Meridian)

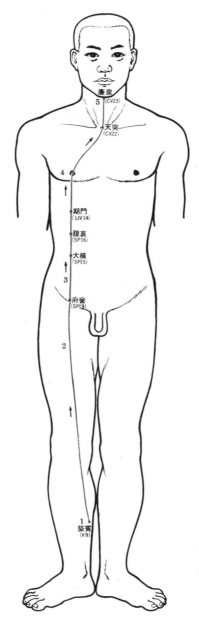

廉泉
5 (CV23)

天突
(CV22)

4

期門
(LIV 14)

腹哀
(SP16)

大横
(SP15)

3

府舍
(SP13)

2

1
築賓
(K9)

Fig. 39 Yin Wai Mai

Chapter 22

Yin Wai Mai
(The Yin regulation channel)

(A) Direction:

Originates from the Leg Lesser Yin Kidney Meridian at K 9 point, then goes upwards along the medial side of the leg and thigh to the lateral side of the abdomen and chest, then ascends to the throat and connects with the conception vessel at point CV 23. (Fig. 39)

(B) Branches:

None

(C) Connected Internal Organs:

None

(D) Connective Points:

K 9 (the Leg Lesser Yin Kidney Meridian)

SP 13, SP 15, SP 16 (the Greater Yin Spleen Meridian)

Liv 14 (the Leg Absolute Yin Liver Meridian)

CV 22, CV 23 (the Conception Vessel Meridian)

Chapter 23

The commonly used strange acupuncture points

1. **Yin-Tang (Seal Center 印堂)**
   Location: The middle of the line connecting the medial end of the two eyc-brows.
   Indications: Migraine, Hypertension, Convulsion.
   Method of Insertion: Slanting insertion of 0.3 — 0.5 tsun deep.

2. **Tai-Yang (Sun Light 太陽)**
   Location: One tsun behind the lateral canthus.
   Indications: Temporial headache, Blurred vision.
   Method of Insertion: Slanting insertion of 0.5 — 1.0 tsun deep.

3. **Lung-Sueh (Deaf Point 聾穴)**
   Location: The midpoint between SI 19 point and T 21 point.
   Indications: Deafness, Tinnitus.
   Method of Insertion: Straight insertion of 0.3 — 0.5 tsun deep.

4.　**Yu-Yao (Fish Loin 魚腰)**

Location:　The middle of the eyebrow.

Indications: Tic, Paralysis of the palpebral Muscle.

Method of Insertion: Slanting insertion of 0.3 — 0.5 tsun deep.

5.　**Chuan-Hsi (Stop Asthma 喘息)**

Location: One tsun beside GV 14 point.

Indications: Asthma, Urticaria.

Method of Insertion: Slanting insertion of 0.5 — 1.0 tsun deep.

6.　**Hua-To (Hua To Vertebral Points 華陀脊背)**

Location:　There are 17 pairs or 34 points located 0.5 tsun beside and between the spines from the first thoracic vertebra to the fifth lumbar vertebra.

Indications: Asthma, Gastro-Intestinal disease, Impotence, Dysmenorrhoea, Neurasthenia, Lumbago.

Method of Insertion: Straight insertion of 0.5 — 1.0 tsun deep.

7.　**Yi-Ming (Shielding Bright 翳明)**

Location:　One tsun behind T 17 point, at the inferior margin of the mastoid process.

Indications: Myopia, Insomnia.

Method of Insertion: Straight insertion or slanting insertion towards anterio-superior direction 0.6 — 1.0 tsun deep.

8. **Hung-Yin (Torrent Sound 洪音)**
    Location: 0.5 tsun beside the laryngeal prominence.
    Indications: Acute laryngitis, Deaf-mutes.
    Method of Insertion: Straight insertion of 0.3 — 0.5 tsun deep.

9. **Yi-Ching (Emission Point 遺精)**
    Location: One tsun beside CV 4 point.
    Indications: Nocturnal pollution, Impotence.
    Method of Insertion: Straight insertion of 1.5 tsun deep.

10. **Tsu-Kung (Uterus Point 子宮)**
    Location: 3 tsun beside and one tsun below CV 4 point.
    Indications: Irregular menstruation, Endometritis.
    Method of Insertion: Straight insertion of 1.0 — 1.5 tsun deep.

11. **Chih-Yao (Ulnar - Radial 尺橈)**
    Location: 6 tsun above the middle of the wrist crease, midpoint between the ulnar-Radial bones of the back of the forearm.
    Indications: Arm pain, Insanity.

Method of Insertion: Straight insertion of 1.0 — 1.5 tsun deep.

12. **Yi-Shu (Pancrease Locus** 胰俞 **)**

    Location: 1.5 tsun beside and between the thoracic vertebra T 8 and T 9.

    Indications: Chornic pancreatitis, Indigestion.

    Method of Insertion: Slanting insertion of 0.5 — 1.0 deep.

13. **Pi-Ken (Mass Root** 痞根 **)**

    Location: 3.5 tsun beside and between the lumbar vertebra L 1 and L 2.

    Indications: Nephritis, Lumbago.

    Method of Insertion: Straight insertion of 1.0 — 1.5 tsun deep.

14. **Yao-Yen (Loin Eye** 腰眼 **)**

    Location: 4 tsun beside the lower end of the spinous process of the 4th. lumbar vertebra.

    Indications: Lumbago, Gynecologic disease.

    Method of Insertion: Straight insertion of 1.0 — 1.5 tsun deep.

15. **Shih-Hsuan (Ten Declaration** 十宣 **)**

    Location: Tip of the ten fingers.

    Indications: Epilepsy, Syncope, Apoplexy.

Method of Insertion: Triangle needle insert on the point until a little bleeding.

16. **Szu-Feng (Four sews 四縫)**
Location: Middle of the first interphalangeal joint crease on the second, middle, fourth and little fingers.
Indications: Indigestion, Snake bite.
Method of Insertion: Shallow insertion 0.1 tsun deep.

17. **Pa-Hsieh (Eight evils 八邪)**
Location: There are eight points, between the inter-metacarpo-phalangeal joints on the dorsum of the hands.
Indications: Metacarpo - phalangeal joint pain, Snake bite.
Method of Insertion: Slanting insertion of 0.2 − 0.3 tsun deep.

18. **Lan-Wel (Appendix point 闌尾)**
Location: 2 tsun below S 36 point.
Indications: Acute appendicitis, Abscess of appendix.
Method of Insertion: Straight insertion of 0.5 − 1.5 tsun deep.

19. **Tan-Lang-Tien (Gall Bladder point 胆囊點)**
Location: One tsun below GB 34 point.

Indications: Cholecystitis, Colic.
Method of Insertion: Straight insertion of 1.5 — 2.0 tsun deep.

20. **Pa-Feng (Eight Winds 八風)**
   Location: There are eight points, between the inter-metatarso-phalangeal joints on the dorsal surface of the feet.
   Indication: Toe pain, Snake bite, Headache.
   Method of Insertion: Slanting insertion of 0.3 — 0.5 tsun deep.

21. **Hsi-Yen (Knee Eye 膝眼)**
   Location: At the medial inferior of the patella.
   Indication: Knee Pain.
   Method of Insertion: Slanting insertion of 0.5 — 1.0 tsun deep.

22. **He-Ting (Crane Top 鶴頂)**
   Location: At the middle of the upper border of the patella.
   Indications: Hemiplegia, Weakness of Knee.
   Method of Insertion: Straight or slanting insertion of 0.5 — 1.0 tsun deep.

Chapter 24

The commonly used new acupuncture points

1. **Pi-Tung (Nasal Communication 鼻通)**
   Location: At the superior end of the nasolabial sulcus.
   Indications: Rhinitis, Nasal discharge.
   Method of Insertion: Slanting insertion of 0.3 — 0.5
   tsun deep.

2. **Ting-Hsueh (Listening point 聽穴)**
   Location: The midpoint between SI 19 and GB 2
   points.
   Indications: Deafness, Tinnitus.
   Method of Insertion: Straight insertion of 0.3 — 0.5
   tsun deep.

3. **Ting-Chung (Listening clever 聽聰)**
   Location: 0.2 tsun below GB 2 point.
   Indications: Tinnitus, Deaf-mute.
   Method of Insertion: Straight insertion of 0.3 tsun deep.

4. **Hou-ting-Hui (Back of Listening meeting 後聽會)**
   Location: 0.5 tsun above T 17 point.

Indications: Bell's palsy, Tinnitus.

Method of Insertion: Slanting insertion 0.5 — 1.0 tsun deep.

5. **Chien-San- Chen (Shoulder three needles 肩三針)**

Location: There are a group of three needles as following:

A. Chien-yu (Shoulder Bone 肩髃)
Same LI 15 point.

B. Chien-Chen(Front of Shoulder 肩前)
One tsun above the anterior axillary fold.

C. Chien-Hou (Back of Shoulder 肩後)
One and half tsun above the posterior axillary fold.

Indications: Shoulder pain, Frozen shoulder, Hemiplegia, Cholecystitis.

Method of Insertion: Slanting insertion of 1.0 — 1.5 tsun deep.

6. **Chien-Hsi (Health Knee 健膝)**

Location: Three tsun proximal to the upper border of patella.

Indications: Weakness of knee.

Straight insertion of 1.0 — 1.5 tsun deep.

7. **An-mien (Asleep 安眠)**

Location: Middle between T 17 and Yi-ming point.
Indication: Insomnia, Migraine, Palpitation.
Method of Insertion: Straight insertion of 0.5 tsun deep.

8. **Ting-Chuan (Antiasthma 定喘)**
Location: 0.5 tsun beside GV 14 point.
Indications: Bronchitis, Asthma.
Method of Insertion: Straight insertion of 1.0 tsun deep.

9. **Hsueh-Ya-Tien (Blood pressure 血壓點)**
Location: 0.5 tsun beside and between C 6 and C 7
vertebra.
Indications: Hypertension, Shock.
Method of Insertion: Straight insertion of 0.5 — 0.8
tsun deep.

10. **Kui-Yang- Sueh (Ulcer point 潰瘍穴)**
Location: 6 tsun beside and between T 12 and L 1
points.
Indications: Stomach and duodenal ulcer.
Method of Insertion: Slanting insertion 0.4 — 0.8
tsun deep.

Chapter 25
Clinical treatment

1. **Pain:**
   (1) Wryneck: L 7, B 10, GB 20, GV 14.
   (2) Shoulder Pain: LI 15, SI 9, SI 12, T 14, LI 14, Chien-San-Chen (New Point).
   (3) Arm Pain: LI 7, LI 14, SI 9, T 14, T 5, Chih-Yao (Strange Point).
   (4) Elbow Pain: L 5, H 3, T 10, LI 11, P 3.
   (5) Wrist Pain: LI 5, H 5, P 7, T 5.
   (6) Metacarpo-Phalangeal Joint Pain: LI 1, T 2, T 3, L 4, L 5, Pah-Sieh (Strange Point).
   (7) Lumbago: B 23, B 25, B 47, GV 4, Pi-ken (Strange Point), Yao-Yen (Strange Point).
   (8) Knee Pain: S 34, LIV 8, S 35, SP 9, SP 10, Hsi-Yen (Strange Point), He-Ting (Strange Point), Chien-Hsi (New Point).
   (9) Ankle Arthritis: S 41, B 60, GB 39, K 3.
   (10) Metatarso- Phalangeal Joint Pain: LIV 2, LIV 3, Pa-Feng (Strange

Point).

(11) Sacral Pain: B 31, B 32, Yao-Yen (Strange Point), B 25.

(12) Coccyx Pain: CV 1, B 34, GB 30, GV 1.

2. **Respiratory Tract:**

(1) Asthma: L 1, B 13, P 5, GV 14, CV 17, CV 22, Chuan-Hsi (Strange Point), Hua-To (Strange Point), Ting-Chuan (New Point).

(2) Bronchitis: L 1, B 12, CV 17, CV 22.

(3) Laryngopharyngitis: LI 1, CV 23, Hung-Yin (Strange Point).

(4) Common Cold: LI 4, B 13, GB 20, Pi-Tung (New Point).

(5) Hemoptysis: L 5, L 10, B 13.

(6) Fever: L 10, LI 1, LI 4, P 3, P 5, GB 20, GV 14.

3. **Cardio-Vasculatory disease:**

(1) Angina Pectoris: H 1, H 7, H 8, H 9, B 15, P 3.

(2) Shock: K 1, GV 26, L 11, Yin-Tong (Strange Point).

(3) Hypertension: LI 11, GB 20, Yin-Tang (Strange Point), Hsueh-Ya-Tien (New Point).

4. **Gastro-Intestinal Tract and Liver:**

(1) Vomiting, Nausea: P 6, GV 20, CV 12, CV 13, CV 17, B 17, LIV 13.

(2) Hiccough: H 7, P 6, P 8, GV 24, Hua-To (Strange
                 Point).
(3) Peptic Ulcer: S 25, S 36, B 21, CV 10, CV 12,
                 Kwi-Yang-Hsueh (New Point).
(4) Distension of the abdomen: S 25, S 36, CV 6,
                 CV 8, K 16.
(5) Diarrhoea and Constipation: B 25, CV 4, K 16, CV
                 8, B 32, B 33, S 36.
(6) Gastroptosis: B 21, CV 12, CV 10, Hua-To (Strange
                 Point).
(7) Indigestion: S 36, CV 8, CV 10, CV 12, B 21, Yi-
                 Shu (Strange Point), Szu-Feng (Strange
                 Point).
(8) Hepatitis: LIV 13, LIV 14, GB 34, Kan-Yen (New
                 Point).
(9) Cholecystitis: S 25, GB 34, LIV 13, S 36, Tan-
                 Lang-Tien (Strange Point).
(10) Appendicitis: S 25, CV 6, CV 8, S 36, K 16,
                 Lanwel (Strange Point).

5.   Nervous System and Psychiatric Disease:
     (1) Headache, Migrane: L 7, L 10, LI 4, S 44, SI 1,
                 LIV 2, T 2.
         Forehead Headache: S 8, T 23, GV 24, B 2, GB 14,
                 Yin-Tang (Strange Point).

         Temporal Headache: S 8, GB 8, GV 20, Tai-Yang

(Strange Point).

Vertex Headache: GV 20, GV 24.

Occipital Headache: GV 15, GV 16, GB 20, B 10.

(2) Hemiplegia: LI 4, LI 14, SI 18, B 50, B 51, B 54, B 60, T 5, GB 30, GB 34, GB 39, GV 16, S 36, S 40, S 44.

(3) Apoplexy: L 11, LI 1, H 9, SI 18, B 60.

(4) Bell's Palsy: LI 4, LI 20, B 2, SI 18, T 17, S 2, S 4, S 6, GB 3, GB 14, Yu-Yao (Strange Point).

(5) Epilepsy: SP 1, K 1, GV 26, H 7, P 8, LIV 3, Yin-Tang (Strange Point).

(6) Coma: L 11, K 1, GV 26, LI 1, Shih-Hsuan (Strange Point).

(7) Masseteric Muscle Spasm: S 6, S 7, L 7, LI 4.

(8) Trigeminal Neuralgia: S 2, GB 14, S 4, CV 24, LI 20.

(9) Intercostal Neuralgia: S 18, H 1, SI 3, LIV 13, LIV 14, CV 17.

(10) Neurasthenia: SP 6, CV 6, B 31, B 33, GV 20.

(11) Gastrocnemius Cramp: B 57, H 7.

(12) Schizophrenia: B 15, P 5, GV 20, GV 24.

(13) Histeria: H 7, B 15, B 10, GV 26.

(14) Anxiety: H 7, P 6, GV 4, GV 14.

(15) Insanity: SP 1, GV 15, H 7, Yin-Tang (Strange Point).

(16) Excessive Dreaming: SP 1, H 7, Yin-Tang (Straight

Point), GV 20.
(17) Insomnia: H 7, P 6, GV 24, An-Mien I (New Point).

(18) Vertigo: GB 8, GV 24, LIV 3, GV 20, Yin-Tang (Strange Point).
(19) Night Sweating: SI 3, K 7, LIV 2, H 7.
(20) Sciatica: B 23, B 50, B 51, B 54, B 60, GB 30, GB 37, GV 4.

6. **Urogenital Disease:**
   (1) Enuresis: K 3, SP 6, SP 9, H 8, GV 4, B 31, B 32.

   (2) Dysuria: SP 6, SP 9, CV 2, CV 4, B 47.
   (3) Nephritis: B 23, K 3, GV 4, CV 2, K 7.
   (4) Impotence: B 23, SP 6, Yi-Ching (Strange Point).

7. **Eye, Ear, Nose, Mouth:**
   (1) Myopia, Conjunctivitis, Keratitis: S 1, B 1, GB 1, GB 37, Yu-Yao (Strange Point), Yi-Ming (Strange Point).
   (2) Deafness: LI 5, T 2, T 21, SI 9, SI 19, CV 23, GV 15, GB 2, Lung-Sueh (Strange Point), Ting-Hsueh (New Point).
   (3) Aphasia: H 5, Hung-Yin (Strange Point).
   (4) Tinnitus: T 5, T 17, SI 19, GB 2, GV 20, Ting-

Chung (New Point) Hou-Ting-Hui (New Point).

(5) Rhinitis: LI 20, LI 4, L 7, SI 18, Pi-Tung (New Point).

(6) Toothache: LI 4, S 4, S 6, S 44, SI 18, GB 3, CV 27, CV 24.

8. **Gynecological and Obstetric Disease:**

(1) Dysmenorrhoea: SP 6, CV 4, GV 4, SP 10, Yao-Yen (Strange Point).

(2) Irregular Menstruation: SP 6, B 32, CV 2, Tsu-Kung (Strange Point).

(3) Menorrhagia: SP 6, SP 10, H 7, CV 6, Hua-To Point (Strange Point).

(4) Prolonged Labour: B 67, LI 11, LI 4, SP 6, Tsu-Kung (Strange Point).

(5) Poor Lactation: S 18, SI 1, CV 17, P 6.

Index

1. THE ARM GREATER YIN LUNGS MERIDIAN

L 1	(52)	Chungfu	中府
L 2	(53)	Yunmen	云門
L 3	(54)	Tienfu	天府
L 4	(55)	Hsiapai	俠白
L 5	(56)	Chihtse	尺澤
L 6	(57)	Kungtsui	孔最
L 7	(58)	Liehchueh	列缺
L 8	(59)	Chingchu	經渠
L 9	(60)	Taiyuan	太淵
L 10	(61)	Yuchi	魚際
L 11	(62)	Shaoshang	少商

2. THE ARM SUNLIGHT YANG LARGE INTESTINE MERIDIAN

LI 1	(81)	Shangyang	商陽
LI 2	(82)	Erhchien	二間
LI 3	(83)	Sanchien	三間

— LI 4	(84)	Hoku	合谷
LI 5	(85)	Yanghsi	陽谿
LI 6	(86)	Pienli	偏歷
LI 7	(87)	Wenliu	溫溜
LI 8	(88)	Hsialien	下廉
LI 9	(89)	Shanglien	上廉
LI 10	(90)	Sanli	三里
LI 11	(91)	Chuchih	曲池
LI 12	(92)	Chouliao	肘髎
LI 13	(93)	Wuli	五里
LI 14	(94)	Pinao	臂臑
LI 15	(95)	Chienyu	肩髃
LI 16	(96)	Chuku	巨骨
LI 17	(97)	Tienting	天鼎
LI 18	(98)	Futu	扶突
LI 19	(99)	Holiao	和髎
LI 20	(100)	Yinghsiang	迎香

3. THE LEG SUNLIGHT YANG STOMACH MERIDIAN

S 1	(143)	Chengchi	承泣
S 2	(144)	Szupai	四白
S 3	(145)	Chuliao	巨髎
S 4	(146)	Titsang	地倉
S 5	(147)	Taying	大迎
S 6	(148)	Chiache	頰車

S	7	(149)	Hsiakuan	下關
S	8	(150)	Touwei	頭維
S	9	(151)	Jenying	人迎
S	10	(152)	Shuitu	水突
S	11	(153)	Chishe	氣舍
S	12	(154)	Chuehpen	缺盆
S	13	(155)	Chihu	氣戶
S	14	(156)	Kufang	庫房
S	15	(157)	Wuyi	屋翳
S	16	(158)	Yingchuang	膺窗
S	17	(159)	Juchung	乳中
S	18	(160)	Juken	乳根
S	19	(161)	Puyung	不容
S	20	(162)	Chengman	承滿
S	21	(163)	Liangmen	梁門
S	22	(164)	Kuanmen	關門
S	23	(165)	Taiyi	太乙
S	24	(166)	Huajoumen	滑肉門
S	25	(167)	Tienshu	天樞
S	26	(168)	Wailing	外陵
S	27	(169)	Tachu	大巨
S	28	(170)	Shuitao	水道
S	29	(171)	Kuilai	歸來
S	30	(172)	Chichung	氣衝
S	31	(173)	Pikuan	髀關
S	32	(174)	Futu	伏兔
S	33	(175)	Yinshih	陰市

S 34	(176)	Liangchiu	梁丘
S 35	(177)	Tupi	犢鼻
S 36	(178)	Tsusanli	足三里
S 37	(179)	Shangchuhsu	上巨虛
S 38	(180)	Tiaokou	條口
S 39	(181)	Hsiachuhsu	下巨虛
S 40	(182)	Fenglung	豐隆
S 41	(183)	Chiehhsi	解谿
S 42	(184)	Chungyang	衝陽
S 43	(185)	Hsienku	陷谷
S 44	(186)	Neiting	內庭
S 45	(187)	Litui	厲兌

4. THE LEG GREATER YIN SPLEEN MERIDIAN

SP 1	(299)	Yinpai	隱白
SP 2	(300)	Tatu	大都
SP 3	(301)	Taipai	太白
SP 4	(302)	Kungsun	公孫
SP 5	(303)	Shangchiu	商丘
SP 6	(304)	Sanyinchiao	三陰交
SP 7	(305)	Louku	漏谷
SP 8	(306)	Tichi	地機
SP 9	(307)	Yinlingchuan	陰陵泉
SP 10	(308)	Hsuehhai	血海
SP 11	(309)	Chimen	箕門

SP 12	(310)	Chungmen	衝門
SP 13	(311)	Fushe	府舍
SP 14	(312)	Fuchieh	腹結
SP 15	(313)	Taheng	大橫
SP 16	(314)	Fuai	腹哀
SP 17	(315)	Shihtou	食竇
SP 18	(316)	Tienhsi	天谿
SP 19	(317)	Hsiunghsiang	胸鄉
SP 20	(318)	Chouyung	周榮
SP 21	(319)	Tapao	大包

5. THE ARM LESSER YIN HEART MERIDIAN

H 1	(72)	Chichuan	極泉
H 2	(73)	Chingling	靑靈
H 3	(74)	Shaohai	少海
H 4	(75)	Lingtao	靈道
H 5	(76)	Tungli	通里
H 6	(77)	Yinhsi	陰郄
H 7	(78)	Shenmen	神門
H 8	(79)	Shaofu	少府
H 9	(80)	Shaochung	少衝

6. THE ARM GREATER YANG SMALL INTESTINE MERIDIAN

SI 1	(124)	Shaotse	少澤
SI 2	(125)	Chienku	前谷
SI 3	(126)	Houhsi	後谿
SI 4	(127)	Wanku	腕骨
SI 5	(128)	Yangku	陽谷
SI 6	(129)	Yanglao	養老
SI 7	(130)	Chihcheng	支正
SI 8	(131)	Hsiaohai	小海
SI 9	(132)	Chienchen	肩貞
SI 10	(133)	Naoshu	臑俞
SI 11	(134)	Tientsung	天宗
SI 12	(135)	Pingfeng	秉風
SI 13	(136)	Chuyuan	曲垣
SI 14	(137)	Chienwaishu	肩外俞
SI 15	(138)	Chienchungshu	肩中俞
SI 16	(139)	Tienchuang	天窗
SI 17	(140)	Tienyung	天容
SI 18	(141)	Chuanliao	顴髎
SI 19	(142)	Tingkung	聽宮

7. THE LEG GREATER YANG BLADDER MERIDIAN

B 1 (232)	Chingming	睛明
B 2 (233)	Tsanchu	攢竹
B 3 (234)	Meichung	眉衝
B 4 (235)	Chucha	曲差
B 5 (236)	Wuchu	五處
B 6 (237)	Chengkuang	承光
B 7 (238)	Tungtien	通天
B 8 (239)	Lochueh	絡却
B 9 (240)	Yuchen	玉枕
B 10 (241)	Tienchu	天柱
B 11 (242)	Tachu	大杼
B 12 (243)	Fengmen	風門
B 13 (244)	Feishu	肺兪
B 14 (245)	Chuehyinshu	厥陰兪
B 15 (246)	Hsinshu	心兪
B 16 (247)	Tushu	督兪
B 17 (248)	Keshu	膈兪
B 18 (249)	Kanshu	肝兪
B 19 (250)	Tanshu	胆兪
B 20 (251)	Pishu	脾兪
B 21 (252)	Weishu	胃兪
B 22 (253)	Sanchiaoshu	三焦兪
B 23 (254)	Shenshu	腎兪

B	24 (255)	Chihaishu	氣海俞
B	25 (256)	Tachangshu	大腸俞
B	26 (257)	Kuanyuanshu	關元俞
B	27 (258)	Hsiaochangshu	小腸俞
B	28 (259)	Pangkuangshu	膀胱俞
B	29 (260)	Chunglushu	中膂俞
B	30 (261)	Paihuanshu	白環俞
B	31 (262)	Shangliao	上髎
B	32 (263)	Tzuliao	次髎
B	33 (264)	Chungliao	中髎
B	34 (265)	Hsialiao	下髎
B	35 (266)	Huiyang	會陽
B	36 (267)	Fufen	附分
B	37 (268)	Pohu	魄戶
B	38 (269)	Kaohuang	膏肓
B	39 (270)	Shentang	神堂
B	40 (271)	Yihsi	譩譆
B	41 (272)	Kekuan	膈關
B	42 (273)	Hunmen	魂門
B	43 (274)	Yangkang	陽綱
B	44 (275)	Yishe	意舍
B	45 (276)	Weitsang	胃倉
B	46 (277)	Huangmen	肓門
B	47 (278)	Chihshih	志室
B	48 (279)	Paohuang	胞肓
B	49 (280)	Chihpien	秩邊
B	50 (281)	Chengfu	承扶

B 51	(282)	Yinmen	殷門
B 52	(283)	Fuhsi	浮郄
B 53	(284)	Weiyang	委陽
B 54	(285)	Weichung	委中 一
B 55	(286)	Hoyang	合陽
B 56	(287)	Chengchin	承筋
B 57	(288)	Chengshan	承山
B 58	(289)	Feiyang	飛揚
B 59	(290)	Fuyang	跗陽
B 60	(291)	Kunlun	昆崙
B 61	(292)	Pushen	僕參
B 62	(293)	Shenmo	申脈
B 63	(294)	Chinmen	金門
B 64	(295)	Chingku	京骨
B 65	(296)	Shuku	束骨
B 66	(297)	Tungku	通谷
B 67	(298)	Chihyin	至陰

8. THE LEG LESSER YIN KIDNEYS MERIDIAN

K 1	(334)	Yungchuan	湧泉
K 2	(335)	Janku	然谷
K 3	(336)	Taihsi	太谿
K 4	(337)	Tachung	大鐘
K 5	(338)	Shuichuan	水泉
K 6	(339)	Chaohai	照海

K 7 (340)	Fuliu	復溜
K 8 (341)	Chiaochsin	交信
K 9 (342)	Chupin	築賓
K 10 (343)	Yinku	陰谷
K 11 (344)	Hengku	橫骨
K 12 (345)	Taheh	大赫
K 13 (346)	Chihsueh	氣穴
K 14 (347)	Szuman	四滿
K 15 (348)	Chungchu	中注
K 16 (349)	Huangshu	肓俞
K 17 (350)	Shangchu	商曲
K 18 (351)	Shihkuan	石關
K 19 (352)	Yintu	陰都
K 20 (353)	Tungku	通谷
K 21 (354)	Yumen	幽門
K 22 (355)	Pulang	步廊
K 23 (356)	Shenfeng	神封
K 24 (357)	Linghsu	靈墟
K 25 (358)	Shentsang	神藏
K 26 (359)	Yuchung	彧中
K 27 (360)	Shufu	俞府

9. THE ARM ABSOLUTE YIN PERICARDIUM MERIDIAN

P 1 (63)	Tienchih	天池
P 2 (64)	Tienchuan	天泉

P	3	(65)	Chutse	曲澤
P	4	(66)	Hsimen	郄門
P	5	(67)	Chienshih	間使
P	6	(68)	Neikuan	內關 ✓
P	7	(69)	Taling	大陵
P	8	(70)	Laokung	勞宮
P	9	(71)	Chungchung	中衝

10. THE ARM LESSER YANG TRIPLE WARMER MERIDIAN

TW	1	(101)	Kuanchung	關衝
TW	2	(102)	Yemen	液門
TW	3	(103)	Chungchu	中渚
TW	4	(104)	Yangchih	陽池
TW	5	(105)	Waikuan	外關 ✓
TW	6	(106)	Chihkou	支溝
TW	7	(107)	Huitsung	會宗
TW	8	(108)	Sanyanglo	三陽絡
TW	9	(109)	Szutu	四瀆
TW	10	(110)	Tienching	天井
TW	11	(111)	Chinglengyuan	清冷淵
TW	12	(112)	Hsiaolo	消濼
TW	13	(113)	Naohui	臑會
TW	14	(114)	Chienliao	肩髎
TW	15	(115)	Tienliao	天髎
TW	16	(116)	Tienyu	天牖

TW 17 (117)	Yifeng	翳風
TW 18 (118)	Chihmo	瘈脈
TW 19 (119)	Luhsi	顱息
TW 20 (120)	Chuehsun	角孫
TW 21 (121)	Erhmen	耳門
TW 22 (122)	Holiao	和髎
TW 23 (123)	Ssuchukung	絲竹空

11. THE LEG LESSER YANG GALL-BLADDER MERIDIAN

GB 1 (188)	Tungtzuliao	瞳子髎
GB 2 (189)	Tinghui	聽會
GB 3 (190)	Shangkuan	上關
GB 4 (191)	Hanyen	頷厭
GB 5 (192)	Hsuanlu	懸顱
GB 6 (193)	Hsuanli	懸釐
GB 7 (194)	Chupin	曲鬢
GB 8 (195)	Shuaiku	率谷
GB 9 (196)	Tienchung	天衝
GB 10 (197)	Fupai	浮白
GB 11 (198)	Chiaoyin	竅陰
GB 12 (199)	Wanku	完骨
GB 13 (200)	Penshen	本神
GB 14 (201)	Yangpai	陽白
GB 15 (202)	Linchi	臨泣 ✓
GB 16 (203)	Muchuang	目窗

GB 17 (204)	Chengying	正營
GB 18 (205)	Chengling	承靈
GB 19 (206)	Naokung	腦空
GB 20 (207)	Fengchih	風池
GB 21 (208)	Chienchin	肩井
GB 22 (209)	Yuanyeh	淵液
GB 23 (210)	Chechin	輒筋
GB 24 (211)	Jihyueh	日月
GB 25 (212)	Chingmen	京門
GB 26 (213)	Taimo	帶脈
GB 27 (214)	Wushu	五樞
GB 28 (215)	Weitao	維道
GB 29 (216)	Chuliao	居髎
GB 30 (217)	Huantiao	環跳
GB 31 (218)	Fengshih	風市
GB 32 (219)	Chungtu	中瀆
GB 33 (220)	Hsiyangkuan	膝陽關
GB 34 (221)	Yanglingchuan	陽陵泉
GB 35 (222)	Yangchiao	陽交
GB 36 (223)	Waichiu	外丘
GB 37 (224)	Kuangming	光明
GB 38 (225)	Yangfu	陽輔
GB 39 (226)	Hsuanchung	懸鐘
GB 40 (227)	Chiuhsu	丘墟
GB 41 (228)	Tsulinchi	足臨泣
GB 42 (229)	Tiwuhui	地五會
GB 43 (230)	Hsiahsi	俠溪

GB 44 (231)   Tsuchiaoyin   足竅陰

12. THE LEG ABSOLUTE YIN LIVER MERIDIAN

LIV 1 (320)	Tatun	大敦
LIV 2 (321)	Hsingchien	行間
LIV 3 (322)	Taichung	太衝
LIV 4 (323)	Chungfeng	中封
LIV 5 (324)	Likou	蠡溝
LIV 6 (325)	Chungtu	中都
LIV 7 (326)	Hsikuan	膝關
LIV 8 (327)	Chuchuan	曲泉
LIV 9 (328)	Yinpao	陰包
LIV 10 (329)	Wuli	五里
LIV 11 (330)	Yinlien	陰廉
LIV 12 (331)	Chimo	急脈
LIV 13 (332)	Changmen	章門
LIV 14 (333)	Chimen	期門

13. THE GOVERNING VESSEL

GV 28 (0)	Yinchiao	齦交
GV 27 (1)	Tuituan	兌端
GV 26 (2)	Shuikou	水溝
GV 25 (3)	Suliao	素髎

GV 24 (4)	Shenting	神庭
GV 23 (5)	Shanghsing	上星
GV 22 (6)	Hsinhui	顖會
GV 21 (7)	Chienting	前頂
GV 20 (8)	Paihui	百會 ✓
GV 19 (9)	Houting	後頂
GV 18 (10)	Chiangchien	強間
GV 17 (11)	Naohu	腦戶
GV 16 (12)	Fengfu	風府
GV 15 (13)	Yamen	啞門
GV 14 (14)	Tachui	大椎
GV 13 (15)	Taotao	陶道
GV 12 (16)	Shenchu	身柱
GV 11 (17)	Shentao	神道
GV 10 (18)	Lingtai	靈台
GV 9 (19)	Chihyang	至陽
GV 8 (20)	Chinso	筋縮
GV 7 (21)	Chungshu	中樞
GV 6 (22)	Chichung	脊中
GV 5 (23)	Hsuanshu	懸樞 ✓
GV 4 (24)	Mingmen	命門
GV 3 (25)	Yangkuan	陽關
GV 2 (26)	Yaoshu	腰俞 ✓
GV 1 (27)	Changchiang	長強

14. THE VESSEL OF CONCEPTION

CV 24 (28)	Chengchiang	承漿
CV 23 (29)	Lienchuan	廉泉
CV 22 (30)	Tientu	天突
CV 21 (31)	Hsuanchi	璇璣
CV 20 (32)	Huakai	華蓋
CV 19 (33)	Tzukung	紫宮
CV 18 (34)	Yutang	玉堂
CV 17 (35)	Shanchung	膻中
CV 16 (36)	Chungting	中庭
CV 15 (37)	Chiuwei	鳩尾
CV 14 (38)	Chuchueh	巨闕
CV 13 (39)	Shangwan	上脘
CV 12 (40)	Chungwan	中脘
CV 11 (41)	Chienli	建里
CV 10 (42)	Hsiawan	下脘
CV 9 (43)	Shuifen	水分
CV 8 (44)	Shenchueh	神闕
CV 7 (45)	Yinchiao	陰交
CV 6 (46)	Chihai	氣海
CV 5 (47)	Shihmen	石門
CV 4 (48)	Kuanyuan	關元
CV 3 (49)	Chungchi	中極
CV 2 (50)	Chuku	曲骨

CV 1 (51)   Huiyin   會陰

15. SOME OF THE EXTRAORDINARY POINTS:

EM 12 (Shangming) 上明 ：
 Below the middle of the eyebrow, beneath the superior border of orbit.

EM 13 (Qiuhou) 球後 ：
 At the junction lateral 1/4 part of the inferior border of orbit.

EM 14 (Erjian) 耳尖 ：
 At the upper part of the helix.

EM 16 (Houtinggong) 後聽宮 ：
 Behind the root of the ear, same level with the GB 2 Points.

EM 17 (Jianei) 頰內 ：
 On the buccal mucosa, same level with the first molar.

EM 57 (Zuxin) 足心 ：
 1 tsun behind K 1 point.

Appendix

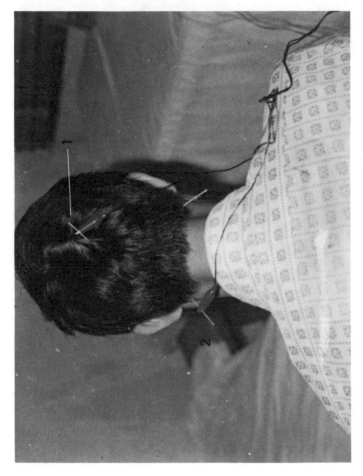

Fig. 40　(1) GV 17　(2) GB 20

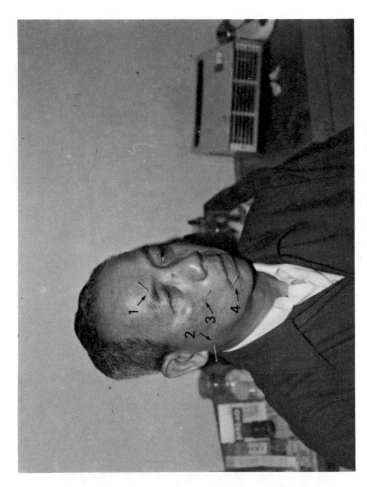

Fig. 41 (1) GB 14 (2) S 6 (3) S 3 (4) S 4

144

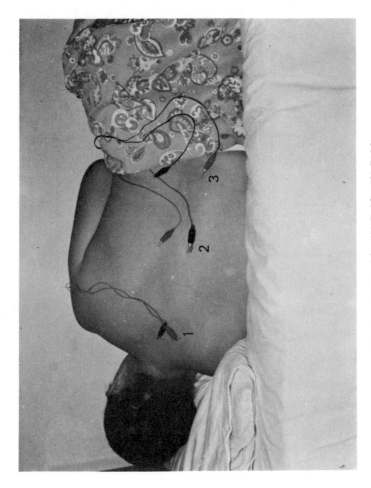

Fig. 42　(1) B 13　(2) B 19　(3) B 23

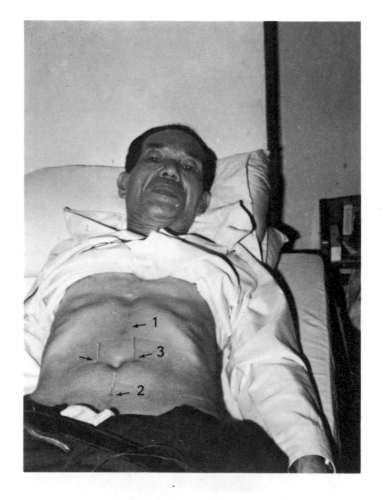

Fig. 43   (1) CV 12   (2) CV 4   (3) S 25

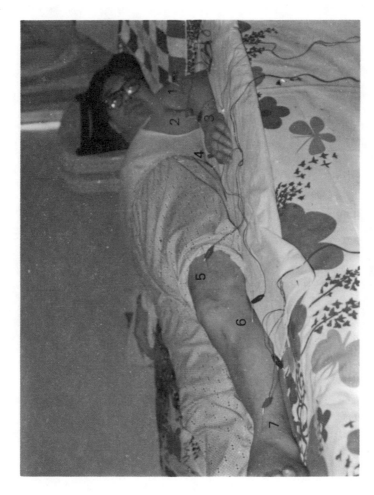

Fig. 44 (1) LI 11 (2) TW 5 (3) TW 4 (4) LI 4 (5) GB 34 (6)GB34 (7) S 41

147

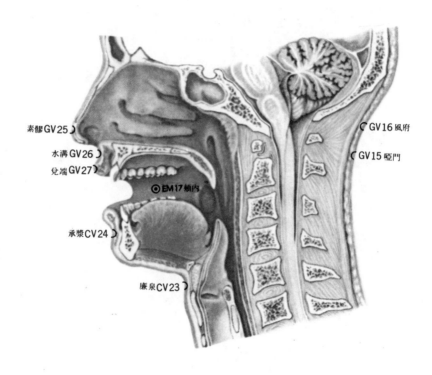

素髎GV25)
水溝GV26)
兌端GV27)
◉EM17 頰內
承漿CV24)
廉泉CV23)

(GV16 風府
(GV15 啞門

Fig. 45   Sagittal section of head region

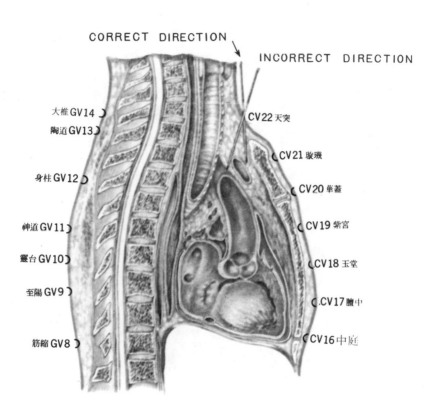

Fig. 46   The angle for inserting needle at CV 22 point

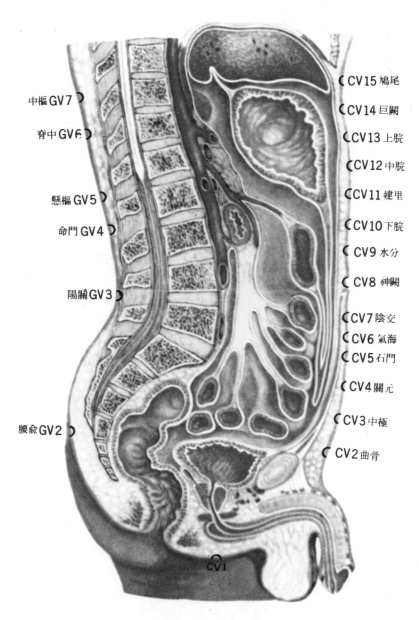

中樞GV7

脊中GV6

懸樞GV5

命門GV4

陽關GV3

腰兪GV2

CV15 鳩尾

CV14 巨闕

CV13 上脘

CV12 中脘

CV11 建里

CV10 下脘

CV9 水分

CV8 神闕

CV7 陰交

CV6 氣海

CV5 石門

CV4 關元

CV3 中極

CV2 曲骨

CV1

150 Fig. 47 Sagittal section of abdominal region.

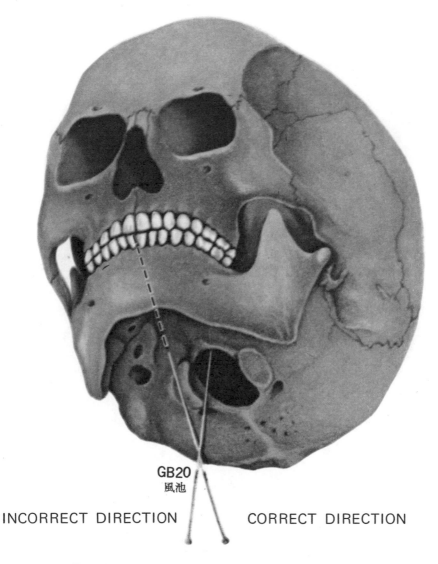

GB20
風池

INCORRECT DIRECTION   CORRECT DIRECTION

Fig. 48   The angle for inserting needle at GB 20 point

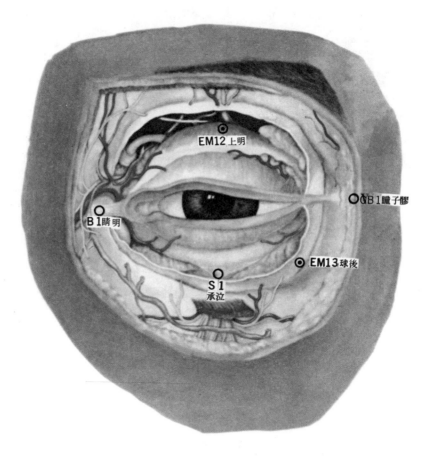

Fig. 49 Dissection of periorbital region

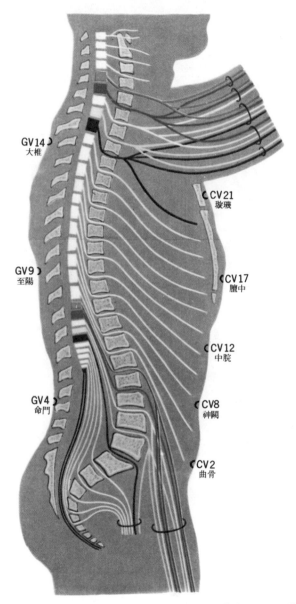

GV14)
大椎

GV9)
至陽

GV4)
命門

CV21)
璇璣

CV17)
膻中

CV12)
中脘

CV8)
神闕

CV2)
曲骨

Fig. 50   The relation of the main points of the conception
vessel and governing vessel to the segments of spinal
cord